Safe and Effective Natural Therapies to Support You Through Cancer Treatment

Jane Collopy
Melinda Hidlebaugh

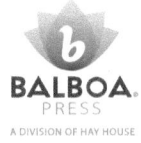

BALBOA.
PRESS
A DIVISION OF HAY HOUSE

*Safe and Effective Natural Therapies to Support You Through Cancer
Treatment* can be ordered through booksellers or by contacting:

Whole Life Naturopathy   Natural Medicine Family Practice
www.wlnaturopathy.com.au   www.nmfp.com.au

Balboa Press
A Division of Hay House
1663 Liberty Drive
Bloomington, IN 47403
www.balboapress.com
1 (877) 407-4847

Because of the dynamic nature of the Internet, any web addresses or links contained in
this book may have changed since publication and may no longer be valid. The views
expressed in this work are solely those of the author and do not necessarily reflect the
views of the publisher, and the publisher hereby disclaims any responsibility for them.

This book offers general information only and cannot consider your specific health
requirements. The authors of this book do not dispense any medical advice or prescribe the
use of any form of treatment for physical, emotional or medical problems without the advice
of a medical practitioner, either directly or indirectly. The intent of the authors is only to offer
information of a general natural to help you in your quest for physical, mental, emotional
and spiritual well-being. In the event you use any of the information in this book for yourself,
which is your right, the authors and publisher assume no responsibility for your actions.

Print information available on the last page.

ISBN: 978-1-4525-2771-0 (sc)
ISBN: 978-1-4525-2773-4 (hc)
ISBN: 978-1-4525-2772-7 (e)

Library of Congress Control Number: 2015902612

Balboa Press rev. date: 08/12/2015

Contents

Foreword ix

Acknowledgements xiii

Why use Naturopathic Therapies During Cancer Treatment? xv

Naturopathic Modalities 1

    Diet and Lifestyle 1

    Herbal Medicine 1

    Nutrition 2

    Homeopathy 2

    Flower Essences 3

    Aromatherapy 3

General Support During Surgery, Chemotherapy and Radiotherapy 5

    Some Helpful Remedies: 6

Common Supplements that Require Caution During Cancer Treatment 11

    During surgery 11

    During chemotherapy and radiotherapy 12

Nausea and Vomiting 15

Mouth Problems 21

    Mouth Ulcers 21

    Alteration in Taste 24

    Oral Thrush 27

    Dry Mouth 30

Loss of Appetite and Weight Loss 33

Gastritis 39

Constipation 43

Diarrhoea 49

Abdominal Pain 55

Hair Loss 59

Skin 63

    Skin Rashes 64

    Skin Burns and Peeling 67

    Skin Infections 69

Pain 71

Anaemia 77

    Low Red Cell Count 77

    Iron Deficiency Anaemia 77

    Megaloblastic Anaemia 78

Fatigue 81

Insomnia 87

Depression 93

Anxiety 99

Stress 105

Psychology, Cancer and Recovery 113

    Psychology and Healing 114

    Psychology and Pain 114

    Mental Imagery in Healing and Rehabilitation 115

    Mindfulness 116

Massage and Cancer Treatment 119

    Oncology Massage 119

    Manual Lymphatic Drainage 120

Appendix 121

    Low Reactive diet 121

Further Reading 125

Endnotes 127

Jane Collopy Principal Naturopath at Whole life Naturopathy.

Bachelor of Health Science (Naturopathy), Graduate Diploma Education, Bachelor of Arts/Bachelor of Theology.

Jane is passionate about empowering her cancer patients to take control of their health by educating them in how natural therapies support their body through rigorous medical treatments. Her interest in supporting people through cancer grew from her own family's experiences of the disease; having the right people involved at the right time can make all the difference to someone's journey through what can be a very difficult time.

Jane is particularly interested in the impact of digestive issues on cancer and how it affects the body's response to cancer treatments. Mood disorders and food allergies are commonly connected to such digestive issues and can make a significant difference to a patient's health and wellbeing.

Jane combines both evidence-based research and traditional naturopathic knowledge to safely reduce the side effects of surgery, chemotherapy and radiotherapy. The naturopathic care she provides during cancer also supports the immune system and raises the body's vitality so that medical treatments are optimised. Jane works collaboratively with other medical practitioners and allied health practitioners to get the best outcomes for her patients.

Jane's holistic approach draws on her background in personal development, education and health science. She is a member of the National Herbalists Association of Australia.

Melinda Hidlebaugh Principal Naturopath at Natural Medicine Family Practice.

Bachelor of Health Science (Complementary Medicine), Adv Dip. Health Science Naturopathy.

Melinda has an interest in all aspects of health and has developed a reputation in the area of natural medicine, caring for patients referred by doctors and allied health professionals. The holistic health care model is an excellent means of managing the needs of Melinda's patients who present with a variety of issues including cancer. Melinda has invaluable experience working within a multidisciplinary clinic.

Melinda uses evidence-based herbal and nutritional medicine, including dietary and lifestyle measures. She holds a Bachelor of Complementary Medicine from Charles Sturt University and an Advanced Diploma of Naturopathy from the Australian College of Natural Medicine. She is currently undertaking post-graduate education specifically in the areas of cancer, women's health, digestive problems, mental health and allergies. Through support, understanding and specialist care Melinda assists her patients through their cancer journey. Melinda is a member of the Australian Natural Therapists Association.

Foreword

In the last two decades there has been a major shift in the way cancer patients approach their recovery. In the past, cancer patients would rely entirely on the medical system for cancer care. In recent years there has been a recognition that patients want more than surgery, chemotherapy, and radiotherapy. It needs to be emphasised that patients are not turning away from medical treatment, nor are patients choosing natural therapies as some sort of rebellion against the medical establishment. In fact, patients always wish to embrace medical treatments for cancer and they see medical treatments as saving their lives.

The difference nowadays is they want to support themselves with natural therapies as well. What seems to be occurring is that cancer patients are choosing to use natural therapies whilst they undergo the rigours of medical treatment. Patients recognise the necessity of decisive, authorative medical intervention for cancer but they also see the sense of using natural therapies to boost their immune system, detoxify their body, lift their energy, and use natural supplements to deal with the debilitating side effects of medical treatments.

Patients appreciate being able to tailor treatments that suit their specific needs and to use both medical and naturopathic therapies that are personally relevant to their situation. Thus patients want to take advantage of all that the medical world has to offer and they also wish to take advantage of all that natural therapies have to offer as well.

Not only do patients wish to combine medical and naturopathic treatments, they also want to be at the centre of treatment planning, and to actively participate in decision making with their medical team.

Research shows that many cancer patients are using natural therapies and they wish to know how best to integrate natural therapies with their medical care. Cancer patients want a better understanding of their illness, their medical options and informed decision making on the role of integrating natural therapies in their recovery. Informed decision making and managing one's own health are important for a patient's sense of confidence and autonomy. Recent studies indicate that patients who have more informed decision making will better manage the impact of their disease on their physical, emotional and social world to maximise the quality of their life.

For this to take place patients will need good credible information on which to base their decisions. So it is very timely indeed that Jane Collopy and Melinda Hidlebaugh's *Safe and Effective Natural Therapies to Support You Through Cancer Treatment* is now available as a resource for patients, their family and carers.

This book will give increased confidence that natural therapies are a valid and useful supportive component for improving well being and assisting recovery in cancer care.

Safe and Effective Natural Therapies to Support You Through Cancer Treatment will also give increased confidence to patients in their ability to discuss with doctors and other support services issues pertaining to their decisions regarding the full range of options for their health care and quality of life by including natural therapies. This book gives clear, easy to follow guidelines for the practical use of natural therapies during the rigours of medical treatment for cancer and for recovery after medical treatments.

Safe and Effective Natural Therapies to Support You Through Cancer Treatment is more than just providing information for patients. It gives doctors, naturopaths and other health professionals the confidence to work together with the patient and their family and carers to develop specific plans for achieving the best outcome according to the expressed wishes of the patient to use natural therapies combined with their medical care.

Greg Connolly
Medical sociologist, Naturopath

Acknowledgements

Special thank you to Greg Connolly for the ongoing support, knowledge and content. Thanks also to Jennifer Burke, Campbell Thompson and Delphine de Jong for their contribution to content.

Thank you to our editors Greg Connolly, Nita Pratt, Dan Duffy, Kim Simpfendorfer, Trisha Grant and Sue Collopy. Your hours of work are so greatly appreciated.

We also acknowledge our teachers, lecturers, supervisors, colleagues and collaborators for sharing their knowledge and experiences with us over the years. To list you all individually would be another book.

And of course our families and friends, thank you for your support and encouragement.

Why use Naturopathic Therapies During Cancer Treatment?

Patients undergoing medical treatments for cancer express a strong interest in the use of natural therapies.

Many people diagnosed with cancer are using some form of natural therapy, however most of them are uncertain why a particular remedy is used, how much they should take, how often they should use it and whether it is compatible with medical treatment.

Many people with cancer are not under the guidance of a fully qualified naturopath and use natural remedies on the recommendation of friends, relatives, books or the Internet. Understandably some confusion may arise regarding the safety and effectiveness of using particular natural therapies alongside surgery, chemotherapy, radiotherapy and other cancer related drug therapies such as hormone treatment.

Naturopaths guide their patients using natural medicines to support their healing and recovery. It is highly recommended that cancer patients are under the personal care of a qualified naturopath, who can monitor the use of remedies alongside medical treatment, support each patient's individual needs and alleviate any concerns they may have. Patients who begin natural therapies find they have a greater sense of control, a more positive outlook, less stress and feel better throughout their medical treatment.

This book is designed as a reference guide to help you discover safe and effective natural therapies to treat the side effects of surgery, chemotherapy and radiotherapy.

Naturopathic and medical treatments can be an ideal combination. Medical treatment will focus on the cancer, and natural therapies can enhance the recovery process by strengthening and supporting the mind and body, and alleviating side effects.

The natural remedies discussed in this book are gentle and easy to administer, and will be a great support for cancer patients during and after medical treatments.

Naturopathic Modalities

Natural medicines are simple, effective and safe when used under the direction of a qualified naturopath. It is important to have advice in selecting high quality products to ensure environmental pollutants, such as heavy metals and organophosphates, have not contaminated them and manufacturing processes have not damaged them. Qualified naturopaths will ensure that your supplements do not interfere with any prescription medications you are taking.

Listed below are several modalities of natural medicine that are recommended for consideration throughout this book.

DIET AND LIFESTYLE

Diet and lifestyle advice is offered to provide simple, realistic and achievable solutions to difficulties that arise during cancer treatment. Recommendations are given regarding food, movement and exercise, sleep, rest and stress management.

HERBAL MEDICINE

Herbal medicines contain a diverse range of active ingredients that improve the function of specific systems of the body. Easily taken as capsules, tablets, liquid tinctures or teas, herbs have a long history of traditional use that is supported by a growing body of scientific evidence.

Tinctures are a potent liquid form of herbal medicine used to treat a large range of health complaints. The dose can alter significantly depending on the strength and extraction process of the tincture.

Tablets are formulated at varying strengths, either alone or in combination with other herbs and nutrients.

Teas are made by diffusing the dried herb in boiled water, and are usually taken at three cups each day.

NUTRITION

Nutritional medicines are used to restore low levels of specific nutrients that are required for the body to maintain optimal functioning. Cancer and its conventional treatment can diminish appetite, leading to an inadequate supply of nutrients. Absorption of nutrients through the digestive system is also challenged and there is an increased requirement of certain nutrients due to high stress levels and increased demands on the immune system. Current food production practices and enhanced farming methods also contribute to a general depletion of nutrients in the food supply. Naturopaths determine the need for therapeutic supplementation, dietary changes and treatment of digestive function by collating signs, symptoms and a range of diagnostic tests.

HOMEOPATHY

Homeopathy aims to trigger the body's natural healing processes using highly diluted substances given as drops or small pills (pillules). It works on a principle that "like cures like." For example, the remedy coffea, which is made from coffee, is effective in relieving sleeplessness and agitation that is caused by drinking coffee. Therefore, the correct remedy is that which best reflects the symptoms experienced by the patient. Please see your naturopath to establish which remedy you need at any particular time.

Low dose homeopathics (6x, 12x and 12c) are safe and effective to use, and can be taken up to four times throughout the day. Only use higher potencies under direction of your naturopath or homeopath. If no improvement after three or four doses, consult your naturopath or homeopath.

FLOWER ESSENCES

The essences of flowers are traditionally used for emotional concerns, such as worry, apprehension, hopelessness, guilt and irritability. The state of our emotions has a major effect on how well we cope with stress and illness. Flower essences can be taken individually or combined with other flower essences. The best ongoing results are achieved by taking four drops four times a day. Four drops of these remedies can also be taken as a single dose, as they do take effect immediately.

AROMATHERAPY

Aromatherapy is the use of essential oils and is part of botanical medicine. Essential oils are extracted from plant material and when prescribed correctly can be used internally and externally to promote health and wellbeing. As essential oils are very potent, only drop doses are used internally, under the supervision of a naturopath.

General Support During Surgery, Chemotherapy and Radiotherapy

Naturopathy specialises in improving the health and vitality of the whole person. This improves the body's capacity to adapt to the significant challenges of cancer by improving the body's ability to make energy and strengthening the body's nervous system and immune system. More specifically, naturopathic treatment can enhance the immune system before surgery, improving wound healing and reducing the risk of infections occurring after surgery. In the lead up to chemotherapy and radiotherapy, supporting the function of the digestive system and liver can improve the body's capacity to eliminate drugs in an efficient and timely manner without reducing their effectiveness in attacking cancer cells. There are also a range of supplements that enhance the effectiveness of chemotherapy and radiotherapy.

The potential for natural medicines to interact with medications and cause adverse reactions does need to be considered. Research is continuously being undertaken to assess the interactions between cancer drugs and natural medicines. Safety and effectiveness are the most important considerations when deciding on supplementation, and advice from your naturopath is essential before combining natural therapies with surgery, chemotherapy and radiotherapy.

SOME HELPFUL REMEDIES:

Slippery elm bark powder soothes and reduces inflammation of the gut lining (including the oesophagus, stomach, small intestine and bowel). This improves the gut's overall function and specifically reduces any diarrhoea that results from chemotherapy or radiotherapy.[1]

Glutamine reduces inflammation and damage to the gut lining caused by treatment. This builds greater gut tolerance to chemotherapy and radiotherapy, allowing these to continue without the need for as many rest days. Less damage to the gut lining also means better absorption of nutrients and less diarrhoea, resulting in better health and less weight loss across the course of treatment.[2] Glutamine can also reduce peripheral neuropathy caused by chemotherapy.[3]

Fish oil has been shown to improve the effectiveness of chemotherapy, increase survival rates during cancer treatment, and protect muscles from wasting away.[4] Studies have shown fish oil can increase the sensitivity of cancer cells to chemotherapy, whilst protecting healthy cells from damage.[5] Preliminary research suggests fish oil specifically protects bone cells from being damaged by chemotherapy.[6]

There are significant variations in the quality and safety of fish oil products available to the general public. Check with your naturopath to ensure you have high quality fish oil that contains the lowest possible mercury level, and has been protected from oxidative damage during processing and storage.

Including fish oil through the diet can reduce the amount of supplemental fish oil required. Choose oily fish such as sardines, salmon, tuna, mackerel, herring, swordfish, rainbow trout, oysters and mussels. It is important to be aware that fish vary greatly in their content of active omega 3 fatty acids; EPA and DHA. They also vary in their mercury content (which can be damaging if consuming fish frequently), and the risk of toxic contamination from waterways. See your naturopath to establish the best selection of fish available to you.

It is important to note that the omega 3 fatty acids found in fish oil are difficult to acquire from a vegetarian diet. Eggs are a reasonable source of DHA, but have very little EPA.[7] Other foods such as flaxseed, flaxseed oil, soy, walnuts and green leafy vegetables do have precursors to both EPA and DHA,[8] but conversion into their active forms is extremely low. These vegetarian sources will therefore not have the same benefits as including fish or fish oil. Vegetarians are still advised to include vegetarian sources in their diet to get what benefit they can.[9]

Folate in its activated form (folinic acid) protects from chemotherapy-induced bone loss.[10] Studies show it can also decrease the occurrence of side effects from methotrexate.[11]

St Mary's thistle protects against chemotherapy-induced toxicity to both the liver and heart muscle.[12] St Mary's thistle also increases sensitivity of cancer cells to chemotherapy.[13]

Indole-3-carbinol increases the sensitivity of cancer cells to chemotherapy.[14] It also enhances the effect of hormone therapies, such as tamoxifen, in reducing the return of cancer.[15] Indole-3-carbinol is found in the cruciferous vegetables (especially broccoli) and can be taken as a supplement.

Black cohosh stimulates the death of breast cancer cells, [16] and reduces the return of breast cancer, even in cases of oestrogen-dependant cancer tumours.[17] Its safety profile is good, with only single reports of toxicity, which were inconclusive and related to adulterated preparations of the herb.[18] Avoid use during chemotherapy however, as black cohosh may become toxic to the liver when combined with drugs that are themselves toxic to the liver.[19]

Antioxidants can have significant benefits during chemotherapy and radiotherapy, reducing toxicity and side effects, protecting healthy cells and improving the effectiveness of the chemotherapy.[20] Antioxidants work by reducing oxidative damage from free radicals in the body. This is important, as chemotherapy and radiotherapy reduce our normal supply of antioxidants. It is important to be aware that some cancer treatments work by causing oxidative damage to the cancer cells;[21] some antioxidants can interfere with this process and reduce the effect of the cancer treatment. On the other hand, some antioxidants improve the effect of chemotherapy and actually protect healthy cells.[22] Therefore it is essential to only use antioxidants under the supervision of your naturopath or oncologist to ensure you are taking those that will benefit you without affecting other treatments.

Mushrooms are known for their immune stimulating effects. Turkey tail mushroom supplements improve the effect of medical cancer treatments, and protect the body from tumour growth.[23] Other mushrooms such as reishi, shiitake and maiitake are also useful, although more research is needed to show their effectiveness.

Arabinoxylan compound has been shown to increase sensitivy of breast cancer cells to chemotherapy. The compound is derived from rice bran and is activated by a shiitake mushroom extract.[24]

Astragalus supports the immune system, increases the effect of chemotherapy and radiotherapy, and reduces their side effects.[25] It should not be taken during the acute stages of an infection.

Green tea improves the effect of chemotherapy and radiotherapy, as well as enhancing targeted hormone treatment in breast and prostate cancer.[26] It also reduces the side effects of chemotherapy and radiotherapy. Be aware that green tea can reduce the bioavailability of some cancer drugs[27] and therefore it is essential to discuss your specific treatment with your naturopath.

Soy food and soy milk are protective against cancer.[28] Whole soy foods such as soy milk, tofu, soy textured protein foods and soy flour have the most protective effects, as compared to soy supplements made from soy isolates.[29] Choose soy products that are made from whole soybeans rather than those that come from genetically modified (GM) crops or isolated soy extracts. The research suggests a dosage of 11 grams each day is optimal, which is equivalent to about one glass of soy milk or half a cup of tofu.[30] In these amounts, soy is safe for cancer patients to consume.[31] Higher amounts of soy, such as 1 litre of soy milk or 2 cups of tofu per day, may be detrimental to the general health of cancer patients who also have low thyroid function, so should be avoided.

Soy also increases the sensitivity of cancer cells to chemotherapy and radiotherapy, and reduces the side effects of chemotherapy.[32] It also increases the protective effect of Tamoxifen and other anti-oestrogen medications, [33] and reduces their side effects, including hot flushes, night sweats, mood changes, skin and mucous membrane dryness.[34]

Common Supplements that Require Caution During Cancer Treatment

Many patients are already taking a range of supplements before they get cancer and wish to continue them whilst undergoing cancer treatment. These supplements may not be particularly indicated for treating a side effect from cancer treatment, but caution still needs to be taken to ensure they are safe to remain on during treatment. Here is a brief outline of some commonly taken supplements that can raise concerns during cancer treatment. In addition, remember that each chemotherapy and radiotherapy regime is unique, and your naturopath and oncologist should check all supplements taken during treatment for interactions.

DURING SURGERY

The main concern regarding the use of natural supplements before and after surgery is their theoretical potential to increase bleeding. This risk is greater for those with low blood platelet counts caused by cancer or chemotherapy. Common practice is to stop using herbs and nutritionals that are thought to reduce clotting or stimulate blood flow before surgery.[35]

Garlic in large amounts of more than 4-5g per day should be avoided.[36]

Ginger in large amounts of more than 6-10g per day should be avoided.

Vitamin E in doses over 400IU per day should be avoided.[37]

Fish oil has been investigated for increasing the risk of bleeding during surgery. The research indicates that up to 3 grams per day of fish oil does not increase the risk of bleeding during surgery.[38]

DURING CHEMOTHERAPY AND RADIOTHERAPY

A range of herbs have the potential to significantly change the activity of drugs in the body. St John's Wort contains an ingredient called hyperforin that reduces the effect of many chemotherapy drugs.[39] Some standardized extracts of St John's Wort have low hyperforin content and therefore may avoid this problem. Other herbs such as schisandra, goldenseal,[40] berberine, garlic, ginkgo, echinacea, panax ginseng, devil's claw, feverfew, peppermint oil, eucalyptus oil, red clover, valerian, kava and grapefruit juice[41] can also affect liver detoxification pathways and can therefore theoretically remove some chemotherapy drugs from the body too quickly, reducing their potential effectivness. Black cohosh and kava can become toxic to the liver if combined with chemotherapy drugs that are themselves toxic to the liver.[42] Herbs also have the potential to bind and inactivate specific chemotherapeutic drugs, such as when combining green tea with the drug bortezomib.[43] As chemotherapy drugs continue to work in the body after the treatment is given, these interactions may continue for days after. It is important to discuss these potential interactions with your naturopath and oncologist before taking alongside chemotherapy or radiotherapy.

Some nutritional supplements may also interfere with particular chemotherapy and radiation treatments, however the benefits need to be weighed against the specific risks. Studies do suggest that N-acetyl cysteine may block the effectiveness of platinum-based medications,[44] and alpha lipoic acid may interfere with the effectiveness of radiotherapy. There are concerns that glucosamine may reduce the effect of some chemotherapy drugs such as etoposide, doxorubicin and teniposide.[45] Despite their potential in assisting chemotherapy patients, quercetin and high dose co-enzyme Q10 can also interfere with the anti-tumour activity of some chemotherapy drugs. Vitamin E is also thought to reduce the effectiveness of radiotherapy.[46]

Considering the above information, and ongoing research into this area, it is imperative that you consult your naturopath and medical team to ensure you do not inadvertantly take herbs or nutrients that are likely to interfere with your particular cancer treatment. Under the guidance of a qualified naturopath, herbal and nutritional supplements can safely make a significant and positive difference both to the outcome of your medical treatment and your quality of life during it.

Nausea and Vomiting

Nausea and vomiting can result from chemotherapy. The degree of symptoms varies widely between individuals; some people will have none or very minor nausea and vomiting in the day or two after treatment, whilst others will have it constantly throughout their treatment period and for some time after.

The severity of nausea and vomiting can be related to the type of cancer (e.g stomach and oesophageal) or the type of chemotherapy drugs used in treatment. The symptoms may occur within 24 hours of chemotherapy and are often at their strongest two to three days after. Please check with your health care professional if vomiting is ongoing as you may require hospitalisation to increase body fluids.

The cause of the nausea may need to be addressed separately. If you feel nauseous prior to chemotherapy it may be because of anxiety.

There are many natural remedies to assist with nausea and vomiting. You may use these on their own or combine them for maximum effect.

Diet And Lifestyle

Eating when feeling nauseous is easier said than done, however with some planning this obstacle can be overcome. It is important to keep eating to recover your strength, and the best approach is to implement certain measures to reduce the size of the task.

Reduce the size of meals by having small snacks or meals frequently. Have a small meal every two or three hours rather than attempting three larger meals. This can be done by dividing your meals into two and eating the second half a couple of hours after the first.

Avoid heavy, rich, creamy foods that are difficult to digest. Choose meals that are easy to eat and break down, such as soups, salads, steamed vegetables and casseroles.

Remember to include plenty of lean protein to help maintain immune function; select a variety of red and white meats, eggs, tofu, nuts and seeds. Meats can be more easily digested as broths, casseroles and mince, and nuts and seeds can be soaked for a couple of hours to soften. If the smell of food causes nausea, try meals that are cold or at room temperature. Protein powder can be an easy way to increase your daily protein requirements; choose rice, soy or pea based formula if whey protein powders are too difficult to digest or if you have a dairy allergy or intolerance.

Use organic meat, eggs, legumes and grains if available, as they are free from hormones, antibiotics and chemicals.

Before chemotherapy treatment only eat a light meal. If you feel nauseous during chemotherapy then try to eat a couple of hours before treatment starts.

For nausea that starts first thing in the morning, try to eat something before rising from bed; keeping some crackers beside the bed can help with this.

Eat your meals slowly to allow for good digestion. Avoid drinking too many fluids with your meal as they reduce your stomach acid's ability to break down food effectively. Avoid caffeinated drinks as these stimulate the gut via the nervous system. Apple and grape juice are often well tolerated.

Rest after eating, but try to avoid lying flat for an hour after finishing a meal. Many people find relaxation or breathing techniques can be very helpful when experiencing nausea, while some find the distraction of company, music or watching television beneficial.

Herbal Medicine

A number of herbs are helpful in reducing nausea, gastric acidity, "anxious stomach", flatulence and cramping. They can be used individually or blended, and are taken as a liquid tincture, tablet or tea. Use under supervision of your naturopath.

Tincture doses are specific to each individual herb and can alter significantly depending on the strength and extraction process of the tincture.

Tablets are formulated at varying strengths, either alone or in combination with other herbs and nutrients.

Teas are made by diffusing the dried herb in boiled water, and are usually taken at three cups each day.

Lemon balm settles an anxious stomach, reduces bloating and flatulence, assists sleep and reduces fever. Lemon balm also has antimicrobial and antiviral properties.

Ginger reduces nausea, bloating, flatulence, indigestion, gut spasms, pain and inflammation of the stomach lining. It is also used to reduce motion sickness, strengthen digestion and improve appetite. Rheumatic pains of arthritis can also be relieved by ginger.

Peppermint reduces stomach cramps, vomiting, bloating, flatulence and an anxious stomach. Peppermint is also good for relaxation.

Meadowsweet is a natural antacid, reduces inflammation and tones the stomach lining.

Black horehound reduces an anxious stomach, nausea, vomiting, motion sickness and indigestion.

Chamomile settles an anxious stomach, reduces gut cramping, spasms and inflammation of the stomach lining.

There are combination herbal preparations available that are effective for a range of stomach and lower gut complaints.

Nutrition

Specific nutrients can be used to support certain functions in the body. Although many of these are present in the diet, much higher levels of particular nutrients may be required.

Vitamin B6 can assist significantly in reducing nausea severity. This is best taken in small, divided doses across the day. Improvements can be seen in two to three days. Be aware that B6 it is often included in a number of supplements. Ask your naturopath which dose you require for safe and effective results.

Homeopathy

Select one of the following remedies. Take two drops or pillules up to four times per day or until symptoms start to improve. Stop taking the remedy once symptoms resolve. If the symptoms return, take the remedy again until symptoms improve.

Ars alb for nausea, retching and vomiting, often from the slightest food or drink, burning pain in the stomach, vomiting with diarrhoea, when fruit doesn't agree (especially watery fruit), when you cannot bear the sight or smell of food, have great thirst and drink small amounts frequently, have heartburn or burping. Ars alb is good for people who are generally chilly, whose symptoms are worse after midnight and better for heat and having their head elevated.

Ipecac for persistent nausea and vomiting especially after foods that are not easy to digest such as cakes and breads. For vomiting when the tongue remains clean and there is a lot of saliva. For nausea resulting from looking at moving objects and for symptoms that are worse when lying down.

Nux vom for nausea and vomiting caused by over indulging in food. Nux vom is also indicated if you have a sour taste in mouth, want to vomit but cannot. It is used for constipation, abdominal bloating and pain that lasts for hours after eating. It is also for a sensitive stomach, great hunger and irritability. Symptoms that indicate that nux vom is the correct remedy tend to be worse in the morning, after spices and stimulants, cold weather and better during the evening when resting, or in damp wet weather.

Verat alb is indicated when there is profuse, copious and violent nausea and vomiting, but is accompanied by great hunger. It's used especially when you crave cold water but vomit it immediately after drinking it. You may crave fruit, juicy foods, cold foods or ice. Other indicators are feeling the cold or having cold sweats. Verat alb is used when any of your symptoms are worse for moving and drinking, are worse at night time, or are better for warm weather or walking around.

If unsure which remedy to choose, combination preparations are available or see your naturopath.

Aromatherapy

Essential oils are complex substances that possess a vibrant quality and distinctive fragrance. They act on the body via inhalation, stimulating the olfactory nerve. A few drops of the following oils can be used in massage, added to a warm bath or used in a vapouriser. They can be used individually or blended.

Peppermint essential oil has a long history of assisting digestive disorders including nausea and bloating.

Ginger has a warming action and is used for nausea, stress and anxiety.

Fennel is taken for nausea with indigestion and bowel cramps. Fennel is used in Chinese medicine for invigorating the digestive system with its dry, warming qualities.

Mouth Problems

MOUTH ULCERS

During chemotherapy and radiotherapy, the cells lining the mouth are susceptible to damage and infection, leaving the lining ulcerated and painful. If this causes insufficient food intake, nutritional status can be compromised, which further challenges the capacity of non-cancerous cells to heal. Generally speaking, these problems worsen with additional cycles of chemotherapy or when chemotherapy is administered at the same time as radiotherapy.

Diet And Lifestyle

Dental checks are advisable before treatment begins to reduce the risk of infection in the mouth. Good oral hygiene throughout treatment will also reduce the risk of mouth ulcers developing. Avoid toothpaste that contains sodium lauryl sulphate.

To support the immune system, reduce highly refined carbohydrates and sugary foods. Increase almonds, walnuts, pumpkin seeds and seafood, as these foods are high in zinc. The zinc in these foods improves immunity and the ability of the cells that line the mouth to heal.

Maintain good nutritional status to reduce the risk of developing mouth ulcers.

Herbal Medicine

Herbs can be added to water to make an effective mouth wash to heal and relieve the pain of mouth ulcers. Add 1ml of herbal tincture to 50ml of water and use to rinse the mouth three to four times daily:

Sage and **calendula** are astringent and healing to the damaged mucous membranes in the mouth. These may also be taken as teas three times daily.

Kava is an anaesthetic to the mucous membranes that line the mouth.

Chamomile is antimicrobial, anti-inflammatory and inhibits ulceration of mucosal tissue.

Myrrh heals the mucous membranes of the mouth, is anti-inflammatory and relieves pain.

Manuka essential oil reduces ulceration and pain (use two drops only in mouthwash).

Salt water can also be helpful as a mouth rinse due to its antiseptic properties.

Homeopathy

Select one of the following remedies. Take two drops or pillules up to four times per day or until symptoms start to improve. Stop taking the remedy once symptoms resolve. If the symptoms return, take the remedy again until symptoms improve.

Ars alb is indicated for ulcers that burn. You may also have anxiety and restlessness. Ars alb is also for when there is a thirst for frequent sips of water and bad breath.

Merc sol is for ulcers that are yellow with infection, stinging pain, bad breath and a metallic taste in the mouth. You may have a constant desire to swallow, have excess saliva and your gums may bleed easily.

Borax is for ulcers when your mouth has a red lining or is hot with the sensation of being burnt. The ulcers bleed easily, especially the ones on the tongue. They are worse when touched and when eating salty or sour food. Your tongue may be dry and cracked.

Hepar sulph is indicated for ulcers that look like they have fat in them. The pain is worse when you have cold drinks, and your mood is irritable.

Nat phos is for ulcers on tip of the tongue, when you have a yellow creamy coating on the roof of your mouth, sour burping, a sour taste or sour vomiting. You may also have stomach pain.

Nic ac is indicated for ulcers on roof of the mouth, often with cracks at corner of mouth and frequent biting of the tongue and cheek. You might notice foul breath and your mood may be irritable.

Homeopathic mouthwashes containing a combination of remedies are also available.

Nutrition

Specific nutrients can be used to support certain functions in the body. Although many of these are present in the diet, much higher levels of particular nutrients may be required.

Specific nutrients can be used to support certain functions in the body. Although many of these are present in the diet, much higher levels of particular nutrients may be required.

The following nutrients assist in the repair of the mucosal lining of the mouth and tongue:

Vitamin E can be applied topically to resolve mouth ulcers and promote healing.

Vitamin C improves oral immunity by improving collagen production for mucous membrane healing.

Vitamin A improves the capacity of the mouth's mucous membranes to heal. It enhances white blood cell function and helps maintain mucous membrane defences to infection.

Zinc is also required for mucous membrane healing and provides immune support.

Vitamin B supports cellular energy production. Vitamin B12 and folate are particularly important.

Iron is required for optimal immune function and red blood cell production.

Glutamine provides energy to the cells that line the mouth. It also stimulates collagen production for healing and repair.

Multivitamin and mineral formulas combine a range of nutrients. Ensure the dose of each nutrient is adequate to your needs; higher doses of vitamin C are often required. Throat lozenges containing zinc and a range of other nutrients and herbs are also available, and may also help with mouth ulcers.

ALTERATION IN TASTE

Alteration in taste can arise for a number of reasons. A metallic taste can be caused by the response of the liver that is overloaded by the drugs used in treatment. A coated tongue indicates an imbalance of bacteria in the digestive tract. Congested nasal passages can be caused by a depleted immune system. Taste-bud damage can result from some radiotherapy treatment.

Diet And Lifestyle

There is a strong connection between our sense of taste and our sense of smell, so become more aware of the smell of foods to enhance your experience of eating. Foods that look good will also be more appealing, so pay attention to how you present food on the plate. Experiment with different herbs, spices and flavour enhancers such as lemon juice, balsamic vinegar, salt, sugar, soy sauce, tamari and honey.

Rinsing the mouth with salt water can improve taste.

Eating sour foods such as grapefruit, lemon and lime, can also improve taste. Grapefruit can affect the metabolism of some medications, check with your naturopath if your medication is affected.

Avoiding alcohol and caffeine assists to reduce the load on the liver.

Including foods rich in antioxidants can support the liver in preventing drugs from damaging the body. Fresh fruit and vegetables, especially berries, are best eaten raw or lightly steamed to keep their antioxidant content.

Herbal Medicine

A number of herbs are effective in relieving changes in taste. They can be used individually or blended, and are taken as a liquid tincture, tablet or tea. Use under supervision of your naturopath.

> *Tincture* doses are specific to each individual herb and can alter significantly depending on the strength and extraction process of the tincture.

> *Tablets* are formulated at varying strengths, either alone or in combination with other herbs and nutrients.

> *Teas* are made by diffusing the dried herb in boiled water, and are usually taken at three cups each day.

Kava has an anesthetic effect in the mouth, reducing pain and discomfort.

St John's Wort is antiseptic, astringing (tightens and strengthens) and healing to the membranes lining the mouth. If taking medications that are contraindicated with St John's Wort, do not swallow after rinsing the mouth.

Peppermint is pleasant tasting and has an antiseptic action.

Nutrition

Specific nutrients can be used to support certain functions in the body. Although many of these are present in the diet, much higher levels of particular nutrients may be required.

Zinc is required for taste buds to function normally. Zinc is also important for our immune system and healing mucous membranes that line the digestive system.

Digestive enzymes are used to support the digestive system by improving the breakdown of food and improving its absorption.

Probiotics support digestion and immune function by restoring bacterial balance to the body.

Homeopathy

Select one of the following remedies. Take two drops or pillules up to four times per day or until symptoms start to improve. Stop taking the remedy once symptoms resolve. If the symptoms return, take the remedy again until symptoms improve.

Cocculus is indicated for metallic or bitter taste in the mouth or with excess saliva. Cocculus is used when there is nausea, motion sickness, aversion to food, stomach cramps or a strong desire for cold drinks.

Mercurius is given for an unpleasant sweetish metallic taste, bad breath and excess saliva.

Nux vom for a sour or bitter taste in the mouth, especially when there is nausea, bloating, hunger or irritability.

Pulsatilla is indicated for a bitter or greasy taste in the mouth. It is also for a blocked nose, lack of taste for food or when the taste of food remains for a long time.

ORAL THRUSH

Thrush is caused by an overgrowth of fungus called *Candida albicans*. In a healthy body this fungus, along with billions of other microbes, is kept in balance in the digestive system by the immune system. When the immune system is depleted such as in cancer, chemotherapy, radiotherapy or other medications such as antibiotics and cortisone, fungi can rapidly multiply. The overgrowth of *Candida albicans* appears as thick coatings and patches of white on the mucous membranes in the mouth (tongue and mouth lining). These can sometimes bleed and may be painful when touched, as when eating.

Diet And Lifestyle

Certain foods worsen thrush by feeding the fungus. Sugars and refined carbohydrates (lollies, chocolate, cake, biscuits, white breads and pastas) should be avoided for this reason. Fruit can be eaten but not more than three pieces a day; eat as a whole food to ensure fibre content is consumed (avoid fruit juice). It is recommended to avoid alcohol, especially wine and beer, as the yeast and concentrated sugar in these beverages feed the fungus.

Include garlic and coconut as these contain anti-fungal agents. Eating these regularly will support the immune system.

Improving your body's ability to adapt to stress will also improve your immune system; refer to chapter on stress.

Herbal Medicine

A number of herbs are helpful in reducing oral thrush. They can be used individually or blended, and can be added to water to make an effective mouth wash to heal and relieve the pain of mouth ulcers. Add 1ml of tincture to 50ml of water and use to rinse the mouth three to four times daily:

Pau d'arco is traditionally used for thrush, at it is immune enhancing and antifungal.

Calendula is also antifungal. This herb is specific for healing wounds, reducing inflammation and cleaning the body's lymphatic system of old immune cell debris.

Echinacea is well known for its immune stimulating activity. This herb also removes old immune cell debris and is antifungal, anti-inflammatory and antioxidant.

Golden seal tones the mucous membranes of the mouth, is anti-inflammatory and antimicrobial. Its bitter aspect helps to stimulate appetite.

Melissa has antimicrobial and antifungal properties.

Garlic is antiseptic, antimicrobial and enhances microflora balance in the gut, which supports the immune system.

St John's Wort is antiseptic, astringing and healing to the membranes lining the mouth. If taking medications that are contraindicated with St John's Wort, do not swallow after rinsing the mouth.

Nutrition

Specific nutrients can be used to support certain functions in the body. Although many of these are present in the diet, much higher levels of particular nutrients may be required.

Probiotics improve numbers of beneficial bacteria. The strains of probiotics shown to be most beneficial after antibiotics are *Lactobacillus rhamnosus*, *Lactobacillus acidophilus* and *Lactobacillus reuteri*.

Glutamine stimulates immune function, feeds the epithelial cells of the mucous membranes and reduces inflammation.

Omega 3 is anti-inflammatory, decreases pain, boosts immune function and rebuilds the integrity of the mucous membranes in the mouth.

Vitamin C regulates and stimulates the immune system, acts as an antioxidant and reduces inflammation.

Zinc as an antioxidant protects cell membranes from free radical damage, assists healing by building elastic cross linkages and collagen, and is required to build proteins that make up the immune system.

B vitamins are required for immune function and building adrenal hormones that are required in times of stress and immune suppression.

Homeopathy

Select one of the following remedies. Take two drops or pillules up to four times per day or until symptoms start to improve. Stop taking the remedy once symptoms resolve. If the symptoms return, take the remedy again until symptoms improve.

Borax is for when there is a thick white coating and bleeding from the lining of the mouth. It is also indicated when the area is hot and worse for touch and salty or sour food.

Ars alb is for a burning, itching sensation. It is also indicated when there is anxiety.

Sulph ac is indicated when there is bad breath.

Sulphur for when the mouth is red and inflamed as well as worse for water and in the morning.

Mercurius is indicated when you have a lot of saliva, bad breath and a trembling tongue.

Capsicum is for hot and sore patches, as well as when you are worse from drinking cold water.

DRY MOUTH

Also known as xerostomia, dry mouth commonly troubles people with cancer and can be caused by a range of factors including medications (chemotherapy, pain relief medication, sedatives, anti depressants and diuretics), radiotherapy (when salivary glands are exposed to radiation), generalized dehydration or oral thrush.

Diet And Lifestyle

The mouth can be kept moist by rinsing with water every two hours. Adding salt or bitter foods such as lemon can help to stimulate saliva production in the mouth. Humidifiers in the bedroom while sleeping may also help. Keep lips moisterised with a lip balm; try a petroleum free paw paw ointment.

Drink plenty of water to ensure you do not become dehydrated. This is especially important if you have heating on in the main living areas. Minimise caffeine and alcoholic drinks as these will worsen an already dry mouth. Drink herbal teas instead.

Good oils from fish, avocado, nuts and seeds can also help the function of the salivary glands.

Herbal Medicine

Gentian, globe artichoke, dandelion, St Mary's thistle, hops and **centaury** are bitter herbs that stimulate production of saliva. In addition to relieving a dry mouth, the saliva improves food breakdown and stimulates appetite by increasing digestive enzymes. These herbs are ideally taken about 10 to 15 minutes before meals as tinctures or strong teas. Tablets are not suitable, as they do not stimulate the bitter taste buds in the mouth. Use under the supervision of your naturopath.

Nutrition

Specific nutrients can be used to support certain functions in the body. Although many of these are present in the diet, much higher levels of particular nutrients may be required.

Zinc builds proteins for the immune system and protects the cell membranes of the mouth lining from free radical damage.

Vitamin C regulates and stimulates the immune system, is antioxidant and reduces inflammation.

Vitamin B6 is required to make bile (which stimulates salivary production).

Folate and vitamin B12 deficiency can make the tongue dry and red. Blood tests can indicate if deficiency is present.

Homeopathy

Select one of the following remedies. Take two drops or pillules up to four times per day or until symptoms start to improve. Stop taking the remedy once symptoms resolve. If symptoms return, take the remedy again until symptoms improve.

Bryonia for great dryness with a great thirst for large quantities of water. Bryonia is also used for headaches.

Ars alb for dryness when there is a thirst for small quantities of water frequently, especially if you have a tendency to feel the cold.

Nux mosch is indicated when the tongue is so dry it sticks to the roof of the mouth, if the saliva feels like cotton, or there is a dry throat and no thirst.

Lachesis is indicated when you are unable to stick your tongue out of your mouth.

Pulsatilla for when there is bad breath and no thirst.

Loss of Appetite and Weight Loss

Loss of appetite and weight loss often accompanies cancer, chemotherapy and radiotherapy and is known as cachexia. This syndrome is caused by excessive inflammation[47] from the immune system's response to cancer, and increased energy demands of the cancer itself. The more energy expended by the body, the more food is required to replace it, and if this does not happen there will be significant weight loss. Stress, fatigue, nausea, mouth ulcers, medications or liver dysfunction can also cause loss of appetite.

Diet And Lifestyle

To maintain appetite, digestion can be stimulated with bitter foods at mealtimes; try including the citrus peel or juice of a lemon or orange, parsley, endive, silver beet, mustard greens, radicchio, rocket, olives, chicory, bitter melon or cocoa (85% or more dark chocolate).

Protein is most important for rebuilding the body's lean muscle mass and a host of other functions including immune cells and digestive enzymes. Easily digested protein foods include fish, eggs, well-cooked legumes and lentils, tofu, tempeh, nuts and seeds (soak nuts and seeds overnight to soften if required).

Use organic meat, eggs, legumes and grains if available, as they are free from hormones, antibiotics and chemicals.

Smaller amounts of protein are also found in vegetables. Dairy foods are a good source of protein, however some people cannot digest dairy easily. Protein powders can be useful when digestion is very weak; in these cases it is best to choose a non-dairy type protein powder to ensure good absorption. Soy and rice protein powders are available through qualified naturopaths.

Carbohydrates are essential for energy production and storage. Include a range of good quality whole grains, fruit and vegetables such as oats, barley, brown rice, legumes and green vegetables.

Add ginger and turmeric to cooking to improve digestion and reduce inflammation throughout the body. Fish and seaweeds also reduce inflammation due to their high omega 3 content.

Even if you are not hungry, it is important to eat small meals regularly (every two to three hours). Liquid or soft meals high in nutrients can be easier to eat. Try smoothies, soups, porridge, stewed fruit and salad. Keeping some prepared meals in the fridge is a great way to avoid running out of good food options.

To improve the digestion of your food and avoid bloating, chew your food well and eat slowly. Avoid drinking too many fluids with your meal as they dilute the stomach acid that helps to break down major proteins in your food.

The more relaxed you are when you eat, the better your digestion will be. Eating with family or friends can help with this, as can creating a relaxing atmosphere and preparing food that looks appetising!

Herbal Medicine

A number of herbs are helpful in improving appetite and weight gain. They can be used individually or blended, and are taken as a liquid tincture, tablet or tea. Use under supervision of your naturopath.

> *Tincture* doses are specific to each individual herb and can alter significantly depending on the strength and extraction process of the tincture.

Tablets are formulated at varying strengths, either alone or in combination with other herbs and nutrients.

Teas are made by diffusing the dried herb in boiled water, and are usually taken at three cups each day.

Withania is known as an adaptogenic herb that helps the body adapt to physical, mental and emotional change. It is traditionally used for poor appetite and to assist with weight gain.

Gentian, globe artichoke, dandelion, St Mary's thistle, hops and **centaury** are bitter herbs used to stimulate digestion and appetite. They increase digestive enzymes and improve the breakdown role during digestion and metabolism. These are ideally taken about 10 to 15 minutes before meals as tinctures or strong teas (tablets are not suitable as they do not stimulate the bitter taste buds in the mouth).

Ginger and **turmeric** are strong anti-inflammatories to combat the inflammation caused by the immune systems response to cancer. Their warming qualities also improve digestive function.

Nutrition

Specific nutrients can be used to support certain functions in the body. Although many of these are present in the diet, much higher levels of particular nutrients may be required.

Apple cider vinegar increases stomach acid, which improves protein breakdown and stimulates digestive enzymes. Apple cider vinegar is not to be taken if stomach acid is high or if there is an active gastric ulcer; check with your naturopath if you are unsure. If apple cider vinegar is not enough to improve digestion, digestive enzyme tablets may be taken under supervision.

Multivitamin supplements of high quality can help improve nutritional status if you are unable to eat an adequate diet. Some nutrients such as magnesium, calcium, iron, vitamin C and vitamin D may be needed in higher doses than is available in a multivitamin. See your naturopath for an assessment of your specific nutritional requirements.

Omega 3 is required in the membrane of all cells to provide good cell fluidity. This enables more effective docking of all types of proteins at the cell membrane, improving all functions of the body including digestive processes and particularly metabolism of fats.

Homeopathy

Select one of the following remedies. Take two drops or pillules up to four times per day or until symptoms start to improve. Stop taking the remedy once symptoms resolve. If the symptoms return, take the remedy again until symptoms improve.

China is a homeopathic remedy indicated for a decreased appetite that increases while eating.

Calc carb is indicated for decreased appetite when you have a specific aversion to meat.

Nux vom is indicated if you have a reduced appetite with a bitter taste in the mouth and yellow coating on back of your tongue.

Ignatia for when there is complete loss of appetite for food and drink. Also used for cigarette cravings.

Rhus tox is for lack of appetite, particularly when there are hot, burning sensations, aching of joints and muscles, back pain, fever, watering eyes, nausea and vomiting.

Combination formulas are also available.

Aromatherapy

Essential oils are complex substances that possess a vibrant quality and distinctive fragrance. They act on the body via inhalation, stimulating the olfactory nerve. A few drops of the following oils can be used in massage, added to a warm bath, or a vapouriser. They can be used individually or blended.

Peppermint when loss of appetite is due to nausea.

Ginger reduces nausea and is warming to the digestive tract.

Bergamot for lack of appetite due to depressed mood.

Gastritis

Chemotherapy and radiotherapy can cause significant irritation and inflammation of the gastro intestinal tract from the mouth through to the bowel. This gastritis can cause swelling and nausea, and may also be accompanied by burning pains and a feeling of fullness after eating. There are a range of related conditions that require professional diagnosis so please see your naturopath or physician if symptoms do not ease or you have other signs such as black coloured stool.

Diet And Lifestyle

Avoid alcohol, fried foods, spicy foods such as chilli and curry, and acidic foods such as tomatoes, coffee, oranges, lemons, limes and red meat. These can all increase irritation to the stomach lining.

Include small frequent meals, perhaps every three hours, rather than three larger meals.

Medications can aggravate stomach problems, particularly pain relievers and anti-inflammatories. Discuss with your naturopath.

Herbal Medicine

A number of herbs are helpful in improving appetite and weight gain. They can be used individually or blended, and are taken as a liquid tincture, tablet or tea. Use under supervision of your naturopath.

Tincture doses are specific to each individual herb and can alter significantly depending on the strength and extraction process of the tincture.

Tablets are formulated at varying strengths, either alone or in combination with other herbs and nutrients.

Teas are made by diffusing the dried herb in boiled water, and are usually taken at three cups each day.

Slippery elm bark powder soothes the lining of the gut, provides fibre for regular bowel motions, protects the gut lining from stomach acid, provides nutrients to the gut lining for repair and reduces inflammation. Mix one tablespoon into hot water with cinnamon and honey, or add to a few tablespoons of yoghurt.

Licorice soothes the mucous membranes lining the gut, reduces inflammation and the risk of peptic ulcers, supports the body's stress response and encourages regular bowel motions. It is not used in individuals with high stress levels, high blood pressure, and is contra-indicated with some heart medications.

Marshmallow root soothes and calms the gut lining.

Chamomile reduces inflammation of the gut lining, reduces the risk of peptic ulcers, reduces spasm and cramping of the gut, settles bloating and relaxes the nervous system.

Lemon balm calms a bloated stomach, reduces spasm of the bowel muscle, relaxes the nervous system and acts as an antiviral and antimicrobial in the gut.

Meadowsweet is nature's own antacid and is used if stomach acid is too high. Meadowsweet protects the mucous membranes from acidity.

Nutrition

Specific nutrients can be used to support certain functions in the body. Although many of these are present in the diet, much higher levels of particular nutrients may be required.

Glutamine is a food source for the cells lining the small and large intestine. It is anti-inflammatory and has healing effects on the intestinal cells.

Iron and vitamin B12 may be deficient due to gastritis. A blood test can confirm the levels of these nutrients. Deficiency is best treated with a combination of diet (lean animal foods) and supplements in liquid, sub-lingual or tablet form.

Vitamin A is important for repair of the mucous membranes lining the gut and reduces inflammation.

Zinc is also important for mucous membrane repair, reducing inflammation and supporting food breakdown.

Omega 3 builds integrity of cell membranes and reduces inflammation throughout the gastro intestinal tract.

Vitamin C is often deficient in cases of reflux.

Homeopathy

Lyco is used when you have a large appetite but feel full and bloated after only small amounts of food. You may also experience pain and feel sleepy immediately after eating. Lyco is given for a sour taste in the mouth accompanied by lots of flatulence, burping, gurgling sounds, bloating and a distended abdomen. Symptoms are usually worse in late afternoon and when wearing tight clothing around the abdomen. Symptoms feel better after flatulence.

Phos for burning, gnawing pain from the stomach through to the bowel, that is often worse late morning and accompanied by great weakness. You may crave cold food and drinks, both of which temporarily relieve the pain, but are also often vomited back up once they become warm in the stomach.

Ars alb is indicated when you have a bitter, foul or sour taste in the mouth. You may also have a burning pain in the stomach, which feels better for applying something warm to the stomach or consuming hot drinks. Ars alb is used for burping, nausea and vomiting or particularly slimy or bloody mucous. Cold extremities and anxiety are often signs that you will benefit from ars alb.

Nux vom is used for heartburn, flatulence, nausea and vomiting, especially when symptoms are strongest in the morning. It is particularly helpful when vomiting improves symptoms. Nux vom is indicated when you feel worse for milk, after taking stimulants, when you have a headache, have symptoms from being sedentary for too long or from overindulging in food, especially spicy foods.

Pulsatilla is for heartburn when there is a sensation of food lodged behind the sternum, with a dry mouth and putrid taste in the mouth, especially when symptoms are strongest in the morning and there is little or no thirst. It is used for that all-gone sensation in the stomach, when food seems to have no taste or there is intolerable nausea. People in need of pulsatilla often crave open air, feel better for sympathy, having cold food and drinks, or they feel worse in a warm stuffy room.

China is for gastritis with great fatigue, or when you feel full after only a few mouthfuls of food. China is also for offensive flatulence, bitter burping, and having the sensation that food is lodged in the oesophagus or is sitting in the stomach for too long. Used especially in those who feint at the slightest cause.

Aconite is for acute gastritis with a distended abdomen. There may be empty burping or a desire to burp but cannot. Also used for nausea, vomiting and profuse sweating. Aconite is especially indicated when there is intolerance to pain, or when there is great anxiety and restlessness.

If unsure which remedy to choose, combination preparations are available or see your naturopath.

Constipation

It is important to achieve healthy bowel activity before cancer treatment begins, as some of the medications cause or worsen constipation. This involves eating enough fibre and bitter foods to stimulate digestive function, drinking plenty of water, and participating in adequate physical activity. Stress can also cause or worsen constipation. Ideally the bowels should move every day, and each motion should pass easily and feel complete.

Severe constipation can result in haemorrhoids, anal fissures, rectal prolapse or even the need to remove dried and hardened stool with an enema. Professional help must be sought if bowels do not move for more than three days in a row, if wind cannot be passed or if the abdomen is rock hard.

Diet And Lifestyle

Fibre is contained in fruit (choose whole fruit, as there is very little fibre left in fruit juice), vegetables (especially cauliflower, broccoli, cabbage, celery, green beans, eggplant and leafy greens), lentils, legumes, nuts and seeds, dark grainy breads, whole grain cereals and bran. Consume a variety of these foods with each meal and snack to improve your bowel motions. People with bowel cancer are at greater risk of bowel obstruction and should consult their practitioner before commencing a high-fibre diet.

To add bulk to the stool and stimulate bowel motions, add a cup of oat bran and one tablespoon of a fibre supplement to breakfast cereal.

Fluid is most important to soften the stool and help fibre swell. The daily requirement of water is 30ml per kilogram of body weight. Include water, herbal teas and fluid contained in meals (such as soup and casseroles). Drinks containing caffeine and sugar are dehydrating and do not add to the daily fluid intake.

Gentle, daily activity will help bowels move. Choose an activity that you enjoy and engage at a level that is comfortable. Consider walking, bike riding, yoga, pilates, and gentle weight training (under supervision). These can be done outside in the fresh air or using exercise equipment indoors at home or the gym.

Our bowels like routine. Sitting on the toilet at the same time each day or in the same routine each day will help bowel motions become more regular; for example after waking, after breakfast, after exercise or after dinner. However avoid suppressing the urge to have a bowel motion as this can worsen constipation.

Herbal Medicine

A number of herbs are helpful in reducing constipation. They can be used individually or blended and are taken as a liquid tincture, tablet, or tea. Use under supervision of your naturopath.

Tincture doses are specific to each individual herb and can alter significantly depending on the strength and extraction process of the tincture.

Tablets are formulated at varying strengths, either alone or in combination with other herbs and nutrients.

Teas are made by diffusing the dried herb in boiled water, and are usually taken at three cups each day.

Dandelion root tea contains inulin that feeds the good intestinal bacteria, as well as improving digestion through its bitter taste.

Psyllium husk forms a mucilaginous gel with water and is used to bulk and regulate the stool. Can also be used for diarrhoea, therefore is appropriate for erratic bowel patterns.

Slippery elm bark powder is used to bulk the stool, soothe and reduce inflammation of the bowel wall, and feed good intestinal bacteria. Can also be used for diarrhoea, therefore is appropriate for erratic bowel patterns.

Cascara is a bitter, stimulating tonic that helps bowels become more regular.

Senna is a stimulating laxative that works by increasing bile release from the gall bladder, which stimulates movement throughout the digestive tract.

Nutrition

Specific nutrients can be used to support certain functions in the body. Although many of these are present in the diet, much higher levels of particular nutrients may be required.

Probiotics improve good bacteria levels in the bowel and have been shown to lessen constipation. Supplementing is initially required, after which a good-quality yoghurt can help maintain adequate levels of bacteria.

Prebiotics contain oligosaccharides such as inulin, which feed the good intestinal bacteria.

Omega 3 assists with the flow of bile from the liver and gall bladder.

Homeopathy

Select one of the following remedies. Take two drops or pilules up to four times per day or until symptoms start to improve. Stop taking the remedy once symptoms resolve. If the symptoms return, take the remedy again until symptoms improve.

Nux vom is indicated when constipation is exacerbated by overindulging or being sedentary. It is especially indicated when there is an urge to pass a bowel motion but it is ineffective. Stools that are passed are often incomplete or feel unsatisfactory.

Alumina is indicated for lazy bowels. The stool may be soft or hard, but is often in small pieces and is always difficult to pass. Alumina is particularly useful when the rectum is dry, inflamed and bleeding around the orifice. The mouth is often also dry.

Bryonia is for stools that are dry, hard, large, and may appear burnt in appearance. It is also used when you feel general dryness throughout the body, especially in the mouth, and this causes great thirst. Bryonia is well indicated when you feel irritable and cannot stand moving.

Graphites is indicated when mucus covers the stool and also when the anus is painful from haemorrhoids or fissures that burn and itch intolerably. There may be no urge to pass the stool for days. Graphites is used when there is aching in the anus after passing stool. It is especially indicated if you are feeling sensitive, nervous, have difficulty getting up in the morning, or have difficulty concentrating.

Lyco is for constipation with lots of flatulence, burping, gurgling sounds, bloating, and a distended abdomen. There is often a tendency not to eat much. Symptoms are worse in the late afternoon and when wearing tight clothing around the abdomen, especially when you feel better after passing flatulence.

Silica is indicated when stool is difficult to pass, has an offensive odour, the abdomen is distended, and especially after losing a lot of fluid from hot weather, diarrhoea, or vomiting. Symptoms are worse for cold weather and nervous excitement and are generally better for being warm. Silica is very effective when you are feeling sensitive, chilly, or have smelly sweat (especially on the feet, despite them being icy cold). There is often an intolerance or dislike of milk.

If you are unsure which remedy to choose, combination preparations are available, or see your naturopath.

Aromatherapy

Essential oils can strengthen digestion and reduce constipation by relaxing the muscles of the bowel wall. In addition to burning the oils, a few drops of oil can be added to a base oil such as almond oil, and massaged into the abdomen in a clockwise direction.

Mandarin, orange, lemon or **rosemary** will help to stimulate the bowel to move.

Marjoram, rosemary, ginger and **peppermint** will help relax abdominal cramping and tension.

Ginger and **peppermint** are also useful if flatulence is a problem.

Diarrhoea

Diarrhoea can be loose bowel motions or an increased frequency of stools, causing an abnormal amount of water loss through the intestines. Along with fluid loss, the body becomes depleted of nutrients and electrolytes, which leads to debilitating fatigue and weight loss. If the situation becomes serious enough, it can delay treatment and requires hospitalization for intravenous fluids to avoid dehydration, kidney damage and even death. Contact your oncology healthcare team if your body temperature rises above 38 degrees, if diarrhoea persists longer than 24 hours at a time, or if blood or mucus appears in the stool.

Diarrhoea becomes more likely when undergoing chemotherapy or radiotherapy, as these treatments often create oxidation and inflammatory damage to the digestive tract lining. Once damaged, the digestive tract is more vulnerable to infection. Infective diarrhoea can be life threatening and needs to be assessed by a health professional.

Mild diarrhoea caused by chemotherapy and radiotherapy can continue for days, sometimes weeks, after treatment. Fluids and electrolytes must be adequately replaced during this time.

Intestinal permeability or "leaky gut syndrome" is created in the digestive tract from irritation and inflammation of the intestinal wall. This allows partially digested food and bacterial fragments to cross the digestive wall, causing inflammation throughout the body, and can contribute to a variety of conditions including diarrhoea, bloating, and immune imbalance.

Diet And Lifestyle

Large volumes of fluid are lost from the body during diarrhoea, so it is important to increase your water intake. To replenish lost nutrients, include broths, miso soup, diluted fruit juices, and electrolyte drinks. Ensure carbonated drinks are flat before drinking.

A number of foods can aggravate diarrhoea. Food sensitivities during diarrhoea can vary among individuals, but generally it is best to avoid foods that are fatty, creamy, and high in sugar. Beans, nuts, seeds, raw vegetables, and many fruits may also aggravate diarrhoea. Be careful to avoid any known food intolerances such as dairy, fructose, or wheat. Lactose intolerance can develop during chemotherapy and usually subsides after treatment concludes. Stimulants such as caffeine, alcohol and spices can also worsen diarrhoea by overstimulating the bowel.

Choose foods that are plain and easy to break down, such as cereals, wholemeal toast, rice (preferably brown or basmati), cooked vegetables, and if tolerable include skin-free chicken, fish, and eggs. Water-soluble fibres such as whole grains (brown rice, barley, wholemeal pasta) and oat bran are particularly good at soaking up excess liquid in the bowel. Foods high in potassium will help to replace what is lost through diarrhoea, however, tolerance to these may vary among individuals; try bananas, apricots, coconut, avocado, pumpkin, potato, parsnip, spinach and tomato. To further reduce fluid loss, green or black tea with a squeeze of lemon will gently astringe (tighten) the bowel lining. Adding sea salt to food can also help the body to retain fluid.

Herbal Medicine

Herbs have a variety of actions that are beneficial for diarrhoea, including astringents, antispasmodics, anti bacterials and antimicrobials. Herbs with high nutritional content are also helpful to offset nutrient loss through diarrhoea. They can be used individually or blended and are taken as a liquid tincture, tablet, or tea. Use under supervision of your naturopath.

> *Tincture* doses are specific to each individual herb and can alter significantly depending on the strength and extraction process of the tincture.

> *Tablets* are formulated at varying strengths, either alone or in combination with other herbs and nutrients.

> *Teas* are made by diffusing the dried herb in boiled water, and are usually taken at three cups each day.

Slippery elm bark powder soothes the lining of the gut, bulks up the stool, provides nutrients to the gut lining for repair and reduces inflammation. Mix one tablespoon into hot water with cinnamon and honey, or add to a few tablespoons of yoghurt.

Nettle leaf has a high level of nutrients that support and strengthen the body. Nettle leaf's astringent properties make it effective for chronic diarrhoea. It can be easily taken as tea.

Chamomile reduces diarrhoea through its anti spasmodic, bitter and anti-inflammatory actions. It is also antimicrobial to bacteria and fungi, and stimulates the immune system.

Calendula has antimicrobial, antibacterial and antifungal properties in addition to healing the lining of the intestinal wall and reducing inflammation.

Geranium is used to tone mucous membranes in order to reduce loss of fluid through diarrhoea.

Agrimony is a bitter tonic, used to stop diarrhoea through its astringent action on the digestive tract.

Oak bark is a strong astringent used in diarrhoea that is unresponsive to other treatments.

Nutrition

Specific nutrients can be used to support certain functions in the body. Although many of these are present in the diet, much higher levels of particular nutrients may be required.

Probiotics modify bowel activity to decrease diarrhoea by reducing the frequency of bowel contractions. The *Lactobacillus* strain is particularly effective for chemotherapy induced diarrhoea, and *Saccharomyces boulardii* is more broadly effective for diarrhoea.

Glutamine is a food source for the cells lining the small and large intestine. It is anti-inflammatory and has healing effects on the intestinal cells.

Cysteine decreases the brain chemical that stimulates bowel motions.

Nutrient loss and malabsorption of nutrients during diarrhoea can lead to multiple deficiencies. Consider supplementing with a multivitamin and protein supplement when dietary intake is inadequate.

Homeopathy

Select one of the following remedies. Take two drops or pillules up to four times per day or until symptoms start to improve. Stop taking the remedy once symptoms resolve. If the symptoms return, take the remedy again until symptoms improve.

Ars alb is for burning, acrid diarrhoea where the stools are thin and watery. There is often great restlessness, intolerance to pain, and nausea and vomiting from the smallest amount of food or drink. Ars alb is particularly indicated when fruit doesn't agree with you (especially watery fruit), when you cannot bear the sight or smell of food and when you have great thirst and prefer to drink small amounts of fluid frequently. This remedy is good for those who are generally chilly, who have worsening of symptoms after midnight and feel better for heat and having their head elevated.

Verat alb is indicated when there is a large amount of watery stool that gushes out forcefully. There can be colic pain beforehand and great fatigue after. The diarrhoea is odourless and watery, and often accompanied by forceful vomiting. This remedy is appropriate when you have great thirst for large amounts of cold water, a tendency to break into a cold sweat, when the skin easily turns blue from the cold, or if you feel worse during chills or from moving around.

Podo is for copious amounts of painless, watery stool that is explosive, frothy and sputters the toilet bowel. The stool is often accompanied by a lot of flatulence, has an offensive smell and may contain undigested food particles. It is well indicated for when you feel faint, weak and "empty" after diarrhoea, and when diarrhoea comes straight after eating or drinking, particularly summer fruits. The diarrhoea may be accompanied by a headache. Podo is also useful for longer term or chronic diarrhoea.

Aloe is for acute, sometimes uncontrollable diarrhoea, where there is much flatulence and sputtering. The stool is mushy or watery and may have mucus present, but is not projectile. There is rumbling and gurgling before stools are passed, and griping pains in the lower abdomen. Aloe is useful when symptoms are worse in the early morning, when standing, and when symptoms improve from lying on your front.

Crot tig is used for diarrhoea where there is a lot of gurgling and a sensation of water swishing in the bowels, and before profuse, sudden and yellow diarrhoea. This remedy is well suited to diarrhoea during the summer months, from the heat, sun or dehydration. Ironically, the diarrhoea is typically worse for consuming even small amounts of fluids or food, but better for drinking hot milk. Crot tig is especially good for diarrhoea that has pain in anus as if a plug was forced outwards.

Phos works well for diarrhoea that has a sudden onset and when it is associated with great nervous debility, weakness, fatigue and weight loss from other chronic health conditions.

Colocyn is the suitable remedy for diarrhoea associated with strong cramping that is better for doubling up, applying hard pressure to the abdomen, and keeping warm.

If unsure which remedy to choose, combination preparations are available or see your naturopath.

Aromatherapy

Essential oils can relax nervous over-stimulation of the digestive tract, which can otherwise aggravate diarrhoea. Add a few drops to a base oil such as almond oil and massage on the abdomen in a clockwise direction.

Chamomile relieves cramping, relaxes the nervous system and reduces irritability.

Lavender relieves anxiety, depressed mood and insomnia.

Peppermint relieves bloating, nausea and spasm of the bowel wall.

Abdominal Pain

Abdominal pain may be due to cramping of the intestinal muscle. This cramping can be caused by irritation and inflammation from chemotherapy and radiotherapy. Pain in the abdomen may also be caused by ulceration of the bowel, another common side effect of chemotherapy and radiotherapy. For strong pain or persistent pain call your oncology health care team.

Diet And Lifestyle

A "low reactive" diet is listed at the end of the book in the appendix. This diet removes foods that provoke irritation and inflammation in the digestive system. These foods have been associated with irritable bowel syndrome (IBS). See your naturopath for individual identification of food allergies and intolerances.

Herbal Medicine

A number of herbs are helpful in improving abdominal pain. They can be used individually or blended, and are taken as a liquid tincture, tablet or tea. Use under supervision of your naturopath.

> *Tincture* doses are specific to each individual herb and can alter significantly depending on the strength and extraction process of the tincture.

> ***Tablets*** are formulated at varying strengths, either alone or in combination with other herbs and nutrients.
>
> ***Teas*** are made by diffusing the dried herb in boiled water, and are usually taken at three cups each day.

Slippery elm powder soothes the lining of the gut, provides fibre for regular bowel motions, protects the gut lining from stomach acid, provides nutrients to the gut lining for repair and reduces inflammation. Mix one tablespoon into hot water with cinnamon and honey, or add to a few tablespoons of yoghurt.

Chamomile, wild yam, cramp bark and **skullcap** can be taken individually or blended as teas or tinctures. They effectively relieve spasm and cramping.

Chamomile, peppermint, lemon balm and fennel relieve abdominal bloating, distension and flatulence.

Nutrition

Specific nutrients can be used to support certain functions in the body. Although many of these are present in the diet, much higher levels of particular nutrients may be required.

Magnesium reduces spasm of the smooth muscle of the bowel. Long term use of magnesium can cause loss of calcium, therefore take under the supervision of a naturopath.

Glutamine is a food source for the cells lining the small and large intestine. It is anti-inflammatory and has healing effects on the intestinal cells.

Homeopathy

Select one of the following remedies. Take two drops or pillules up to four times per day or until symptoms start to improve. Stop taking the remedy once symptoms resolve. If the symptoms return, take the remedy again until symptoms improve.

Bryonia is for sore or stitching pains that are worse for the slightest motion. Bryonia reduces inflammation of the gut lining and is particularly useful when there is a lot of dryness and constipation. This remedy is well suited to pain that is worse for any jarring or coughing, and for when you are particularly irritable.

Chel is for deep colic like pain or stitches, particularly on right hand side of the abdomen. The sensation of this pain can be like a string pulling or constriction. The pain can radiate to the right shoulder or scapula. Chel is well indicated for pain that is worse for pressure on the abdomen and eating fatty foods, and for pain that is better for warm foods or drinks, including milk. If irritability accompanies these symptoms, it is a key sign that you need Chel.

Colocyn is used for constricting, contracting and griping pain in the abdomen, when there is a sensation of the intestines being squeezed through something. Colocyn is well indicated for pain that is better for bending over double, applying pressure or heat, lying on the abdomen and moving around. It is also well indicated if you feel worse after eating or drinking. Colocyn will work well if you are restless with the pain, or the pain is worse for anger or indignation.

Lyco is for abdominal pain where there is lots of flatulence, burping, gurgling sounds, bloating and a distended abdomen. The pain is worse in late afternoon and for wearing tight clothing, and feels better after flatulence. The remedy is well indicated when the appetite is reduced.

Dios is for severe abdominal pain and significant flatulence. This remedy is indicated when the pain is relieved by bending backwards, standing up straight, moving about in open air and applying pressure to the abdomen. Dios is used when the pain is worse for lying down, doubling up, and in the evening and night times.

Mag phos is used for spasmodic cramping pain of the abdomen, especially if the pain radiates to other parts of the body. The pain is often accompanied by exhaustion, both physical and mental. Mag phos is well indicated when the pain feels better with warm applications and pressure, and is worse for becoming cold or applying cold to the abdomen.

Aromatherapy

Essential oils are complex substances that possess a vibrant quality and distinctive fragrance. They act on the body via inhalation, stimulating the olfactory nerve. A few drops of the following oils can be used in massage, added to a warm bath, or a vapouriser. They can be used individually or blended.

Chamomile is used for inflammation and cramping in the digestive tract, irritability and stress.

Lavender can be used to relax abdominal muscles, relieve headaches and nervous exhaustion, and improve mood and sleeping difficulties.

Bergamot is used to relax muscles, refresh the mind and improve a lost appetite caused by low mood.

Hair Loss

Chemotherapy drugs specifically target the fast growing nature of cancer cells. Hair roots are also rapidly growing cells and therefore the drugs can also damage these cells. Natural therapies provide the nutrients that help hair grow back as soon as possible once chemotherapy treatment has finished. There are also natural measures that can slow down the initial loss of hair.

Diet And Lifestyle

Avoid harsh treatments to your hair and scalp prior to and during chemotherapy to encourage hair strength.

Avoid blow-drying hair and allow hair to air dry as much as possible.

Use a soft, preferably boar bristle, brush and a soft pillow. Satin pillow covers reduce the catching of fragile hair.

Use a natural shampoo; avoid shampoos containing sulphates as these strip your hair's natural protection.

Consider a shorter hairstyle. Shorter hair tends to look fuller, reducing the appearance of hair loss.

Foods high in protein are required for hair growth. Include lean red meat such as beef or kangaroo, as well as fish, eggs and chicken. Vegetarian protein sources include legumes and whole grains such as wholemeal bread, brown rice, nuts, seeds and oats. Protein powders can also be used. Many protein powders use whey protein that comes from dairy. Ask your naturopath for a soy or rice protein powder if you are sensitive to dairy.

Use organic meat, eggs, legumes and grains if available, as they are free from hormones, antibiotics and chemicals.

Nutrition

Specific nutrients can be used to support certain functions in the body. Although many of these are present in the diet, much higher levels of particular nutrients may be required.

Protein is an important component of hair structure. Ensure quality protein in the diet as described above. When the body is weak, digestive enzymes can improve digestion of proteins.

Vitamin A is important for a healthy scalp.

B vitamins, particularly B6, folic acid, B12 and biotin, are important for hair growth. The B vitamins improve blood flow and uptake of nutrients into the hair follicle. B6 is particularly strengthening to the hair follicle.

Magnesium reduces inflammation that is associated with hair loss. Long term use of magnesium can cause loss of calcium, therefore magnesium should be taken under the supervision of a naturopath.

Iron and **zinc** deficiency are associated with hair loss. Ensure levels are optimal to encourage new hair growth. Check with your health professional before supplementing with iron, as excessive iron can damage the liver.

Vitamin E improves circulation to the scalp.

Multivitamins can provide good levels of B vitamins; be sure to take a high quality supplement that has adequate dosages of the particular vitamins and minerals you require.

Homeopathy

Select one of the following remedies. Take two drops or pillules up to four times per day or until symptoms start to improve. Stop taking the remedy once symptoms resolve. If the symptoms return, take the remedy again until symptoms improve.

Phos is used when hair falls out in bunches, leaving patches of baldness on the scalp.

Phos ac is used for hair loss from the head, eyebrows, eyelashes and genitals. It is especially well indicated when accompanied by grief, depression, mental exhaustion and diarrhoea.

Pulsatilla is used for hair loss when there is a sensation of having hair in your eyes.

Nit ac is for hair loss when the scalp is sensitive, and you are fatigued, not eating well and have lost weight.

Thuja is for when there is white scaly dandruff accompanying the hair loss.

Med is used for hair loss when the scalp is itchy.

Aromatherapy

Essential oils can be added to olive oil and applied to the hair and scalp. Add up to 20 drops of essential oils to 100ml of olive oil. Apply and wrap head in a towel or scarf and leave for up to three hours before washing oil out of hair gently with shampoo. Choose from the following oils.

Rosemary strengthens the hair shaft, improves hair and scalp health and improves circulation to the scalp.

Cedarwood is for hair loss resulting from immune deficiencies.

Lavender reduces inflammation of the scalp and reduces stress.

Jojoba resembles skin sebum, is moisturizing for dry scalps and reduces inflammation.

Carrot tones the skin, and regenerates skin and hair follicle cells.

Ylang ylang reduces stress and has a long tradition of use in increasing thickness of the hair shaft and growing thicker hair.

Skin

During chemotherapy and radiotherapy the skin is affected in a variety of ways, including peeling, rashes, burns, skin infections and an increased susceptibility to shingles. Natural therapies can reduce this damage and improve the condition of the skin. Inflammation is the way our skin reacts to irritation, infection or injury. It causes redness, swelling, heat and pain by increasing the flow of blood to the area.

Diet And Lifestyle

Inflammatory pathways are easily triggered by poor food choices. Avoid chemicals added to processed foods, such as artificial preservatives, colours, flavours and sweeteners. Fats trigger inflammatory pathways, so avoid fried foods (hot chips, fried chicken, fried fish, etc), smoked meats (bacon, ham, salami, etc) and saturated fats (butter, margarine, ice-cream, cream, fat on meats and chicken). Alcohol, coffee and tobacco also irritate inflammatory pathways. Those with suspected food allergies are best on a low allergy diet until specific allergens are identified; see the appendix.

Include foods high in essential fatty acids, which act to reduce redness and inflammation of the skin. These are found in deep sea fatty fish such as salmon, tuna, mackerel, sardines and anchovies. Lower amounts of essential fatty acids can be found in nuts and seeds, including almonds, walnuts, sunflower and pumpkin seeds; and in good quality cold pressed extra virgin olive oil, nut oils, flaxseed oil and evening primrose oil.

Include lean protein and a variety of coloured vegetables to obtain nutrients required for skin healing; iron, zinc and vitamins A, C and E. Quality protein includes lean red meat such as beef and kangaroo, as well as fish, eggs and chicken. Vegetarian protein sources include legumes and whole grains such as wholemeal bread, brown rice, nuts, seeds and oats. Protein powders can also be used. Many protein powders contain whey protein that comes from dairy. Ask your naturopath for a soy or rice protein powder if you are sensitive to dairy.

Use organic meat, eggs, legumes and grains if available, as they are free from hormones, antibiotics and chemicals.

Avoid putting synthetic materials on burned or peeling skin. Clothing made of 100% cotton is preferred and expose the skin to open air when possible.

SKIN RASHES

Herbal Medicine

Using herbs on the skin for their soothing, antiseptic and anti-inflammatory properties improves healing and assists in fighting infection. The following herbs can be used externally in a cream, or internally as a tea, liquid tincture or tablet. When applying herbs topically, always test a small area first to ensure no sensitivity occurs. Use under supervision of your naturopath.

Tincture doses are specific to each individual herb and can alter significantly depending on the strength and extraction process of the tincture.

Tablets are formulated at varying strengths, either alone or in combination with other herbs and nutrients.

Teas are made by diffusing the dried herb in boiled water, and are usually taken at three cups each day.

Marshmallow root soothes and heals the skin, reduces inflammation, and is especially good for boils, abscesses and ulcers.

Calendula is anti microbial, anti-inflammatory and heals wounds.

Chamomile has antimicrobial properties and reduces inflammation and itching.

Chickweed reduces itchiness and inflammation, and cools and smooths the skin.

Nutrition

Specific nutrients can be used to support certain functions in the body. Although many of these are present in the diet, much higher levels of particular nutrients may be required.

Vitamins A, C, E and zinc all help the skin to heal by supporting collagen production.

B vitamins reduce skin irritation by regulating the stress response.

Omega 3 reduces inflammation of the skin and improves healing.

Homeopathy

Select one of the following remedies. Take two drops or pillules up to four times per day or until symptoms start to improve. Stop taking the remedy once symptoms resolve. If the symptoms return, take the remedy again until symptoms improve.

Urtica is used for stinging, itching, nettle-like rash pain. It reduces redness, blisters, swelling, and blotchy rashes that are worse for scratching and better for applying cold to them. Urtica is especially indicated when associated with food allergy responses.

Sulphur is specifically used for red skin, which is intensely irritated with uncontrollable itchiness. It is particularly effective for skin that is worse for a warm bed or contact with water.

Sepia is used for scaly rashes that are red or brown in colour. It is particularly effective for people who improve in a warm climate or when wearing warm clothing (although sepia is also used if excessive heat worsens the skin due to sweating).

Rhus tox is for skin rashes that form blisters with severe burning or itching sensations that are relieved by applying heat or showering in hot water.

Nat mur is for dry scaly rashes at the edge of the scalp or in the bends of the knees and elbows. It is well indicated when the rest of the skin is oily. Nat mur is well indicated when the person feels worse in direct sunlight and during or after physical exertion. It is good for conditions that are worse when there is emotional distress.

Ledum is used for swollen, puffy and itchy rashes that are better for applying a cold compress.

Graphites is effective for rashes that ooze a sticky, gold-coloured fluid which later dries and crusts over the rash. It is particularly useful when there is intense itching that is worse for warmth and worse at night time.

Bryonia is used for rashes that appear bumpy, dry and are worse for applying heat and pressure to the skin.

Aromatherapy

Essential oils can be added to olive or almond oil or mixed into a teaspoon of cream for application to skin rashes. Use up to ten drops of essential oils per application.

Lavender is anti-inflammatory, reduces itching and improves circulation to the skin while reducing stress.

Clove relieves pain and prevents infection; only use one to two drops.

Tea tree heals the skin, reduces inflammation, prevents infection and stimulates the immune system.

SKIN BURNS AND PEELING

Herbal Medicine

Using herbs on the skin for their soothing, antiseptic and anti-inflammatory properties improves healing and assists in fighting infection. The following herbs can be used externally in a cream, or internally as a tea, liquid tincture or tablet. For radiotherapy always ensure your cream has a water soluble base, as oil soluble creams intensify radiation burns. When applying herbs topically, always test a small area first to ensure no sensitivity occurs. Use under supervision of your naturopath.

Tincture doses are specific to each individual herb and can alter significantly depending on the strength and extraction process of the tincture.

Tablets are formulated at varying strengths, either alone or in combination with other herbs and nutrients.

Teas are made by diffusing the dried herb in boiled water, and are usually taken at three cups each day.

Greater Celandine taken internally protects the skin from burning during radiotherapy, however must only be taken with approval of your naturopath as it has been reported in a small number of cases to have toxic effects to the liver.

Ginger taken internally improves circulation of healing nutrients to the skin and reduces inflammation and pain.

Turmeric taken internally reduces inflammation and pain.

Calendula can be used internally or externally and will reduce inflammation, clean and heal the wound and soothe the skin.

Chamomile soothes the skin, reduces inflammation and assists skin healing.

Nutrition

Specific nutrients can be used to support certain functions in the body. Although many of these are present in the diet, much higher levels of particular nutrients may be required.

Vitamins A, C and E as well as minerals such as zinc assist skin tissue repair and healing.

Homeopathy

Select one of the following remedies. Take two drops or pillules up to four times per day or until symptoms start to improve. Stop taking the remedy once symptoms resolve. If the symptoms return, take the remedy again until symptoms improve.

Arnica reduces pain and swelling straight after the burn. It can then be followed by one of the remedies below.

Urtica takes away the sting of pain that feels like nettle-like rash. It is effective at reducing itching, redness and swelling and can be used to prevent the development of blisters.

Canth is used for intense burning pain, especially if urtica doesn't work. Canth is effective if the burn is starting to blister, and when the pain is better for cold applications, or when you are feeling particularly restless.

Caust can heal old burns that haven't healed well, relieve pain of scar tissue formation and accelerate healing of deep burns. It is particularly indicated when you are feeling sad.

Aromatherapy

Essential oils are complex substances that possess a vibrant quality and distinctive fragrance. They act on the body via inhalation, stimulating the olfactory nerve.

Lavender essential oil is safe to apply to burns, either directly with a cotton ball, or added to a cool bath or on a compress. Lavender promotes healing, reduces infection, blistering and scarring and relaxes the nervous system.

SKIN INFECTIONS

When the skin has been damaged by chemotherapy or radiotherapy burns, it becomes much more susceptible to infection.

Herbal Medicine

Using herbs on the skin for their soothing, antiseptic and anti-inflammatory properties improves healing and assists in fighting infection. The following herbs can be used externally in a cream, or internally as a tea, liquid tincture or tablet. When applying herbs topically, always test a small area first to ensure no sensitivity occurs. Use under supervision of your naturopath.

> *Tincture* doses are specific to each individual herb and can alter significantly depending on the strength and extraction process of the tincture.

> *Tablets* are formulated at varying strengths, either alone or in combination with other herbs and nutrients.

> *Teas* are made by diffusing the dried herb in boiled water, and are usually taken at three cups each day.

Tea tree oil can be added to a carrier oil for skin conditions; it has antibacterial and antiviral properties.

Calendula enhances skin healing, and can be used as a poultice to assist in drawing out a skin infection. Internally, calendula enhances lymphatic clearance of infection.

Pau d'arco can be used topically in a cream for its anti microbial properties.

Thuja has antifungal properties. These can be applied using a cream or poultice. Apply throughout the day.

Echinacea has anti fungal properties and is used internally to stimulate the immune system to fight infection systemically.

Burdock is used internally and has a specific anti microbial role in cleaning infection from within the skin cells. It reduces inflammation and oxidation, and enhances blood and lymphatic cleansing.

Nutrition

Specific nutrients can be used to support certain functions in the body. Although many of these are present in the diet, much higher levels of particular nutrients may be required.

Vitamins A, C, E and **zinc** assist tissue repair and support the immune system.

Aromatherapy

Essential oils are complex substances that possess a vibrant quality and distinctive fragrance. They act on the body via inhalation, stimulating the olfactory nerve. A few drops of the following oils can be used in creams on the skin, in massage oil, added to a warm bath, or a vapouriser. Avoid using directly on an open wound. They can be used individually or blended.

Tea tree has a strong medicinal aroma reflecting its powerful effects. It can be used in an oil burner or in a cream for fungal or bacterial infections.

Eucalyptus has antibacterial properties and reduces inflammation.

Lavender can be used in a bath or added to massage oil. Avoid massage oil if there are open skin infections.

Pain

Pain suffered during cancer can have a huge impact on wellbeing through its effects on sleep, energy levels, mood, appetite and mobility. The pain experienced differs widely, depending on the type of cancer, medical treatments and the person's pre-existing health, which may already involve pain.

Cancer itself can cause pain by spreading into the tissue, destroying local tissue, or putting pressure on nerves, bones or surrounding organs. Pain may also result from the effect of chemical by-products that are released from the cancer cells.

Pain can also be caused by cancer treatments. Surgery can cause pain for some time during recovery. Radiotherapy can cause burning pains or leave the skin feeling tight and uncomfortable as it heals. Pain can also be involved in the wide range of side effects that may result from chemotherapy treatments.

If you have a pre existing health condition that causes pain, or if you generally have a low threshold for pain, this increases the possibility of experiencing pain from cancer. This is due to the body's complex pain cycle feedback systems; once they are activated, you become more sensitive to other pain stimuli.

Depending on the cause, cancer pain may come and go, or be ongoing and persistent.

All issues of pain should be reported promptly to your oncology health care team.

Diet And Lifestyle

The most obvious way to reduce pain from cancer is to address the cause. This can be done through direct treatment of the cancer, or by giving medications or natural medicines to reduce pain activation and inflammation, or by directly addressing other mitigating factors contributing to the pain.

Reducing inflammatory triggers in your diet and lifestyle can help reduce activation of pain cycles. Avoid any foods you know you are allergic to; see your naturopath for testing to identify food allergies. Increase anti-inflammatory foods such as omega 3 in fish, nuts, seeds and oils, and reduce saturated fats that promote inflammation such as dairy, fatty meats and take away meals.

Herbal Medicine

A number of herbs are helpful in improving pain. Use under supervision of your naturopath.

> *Tincture* doses are specific to each individual herb and can alter significantly depending on the strength and extraction process of the tincture.

> *Tablets* are formulated at varying strengths, either alone or in combination with other herbs and nutrients.

> *Teas* are made by diffusing the dried herb in boiled water, and are usually taken at three cups each day.

Corydalis is one of the strongest herbal analgesics, reducing pain by acting on opioid receptors in the brain.

Turmeric acts on a number of pathways to reduce inflammation, oxidation and muscle spasm throughout the body. It also reduces cartilage breakdown thereby reducing the pain of osteoarthritis, and can reduce pain indirectly as it improves the effectiveness of chemotherapy.

Willow bark is a traditional analgesic that reduces inflammation and muscle spasm. It also relaxes blood vessels, which may be responsible for its effectiveness in migraines and headaches. Discuss the use of this herb with your naturopath if you are also taking blood thinning medications such as aspirin.

Californian poppy reduces pain and also relaxes the nervous system, thereby increasing pain tolerance. Californian poppy is often used to help re establish sleep patterns.

Kava acts on the nervous system to reduce anxiety and relax muscles, improving pain, general mood and sleep.

Jamaican dogwood reduces pain, relaxes the nervous system and helps with sleep.

Devil's claw reduces inflammation and pain, particularly relating to back pain.

Ginger reduces pain, inflammation and oxidation, as well as protecting the liver from the side effects of ongoing paracetamol usage. Ginger also improves circulation, which can help clear biochemical waste from areas of pain, and improves oxygen and nutrient delivery to the tissues for healing.

Hemidesmus reduces nerve and inflammatory pain associated with immune conditions such as cancer.

Propolis is a strong anti-inflammatory, which is particularly effective at fighting infectious agents in painful joints.

Nutrition

Specific nutrients can be used to support certain functions in the body. Although many of these are present in the diet, much higher levels of particular nutrients may be required.

Fish oil has multiple anti-inflammatory actions in the body, relieving pain as well as supporting immune function and reducing cachexia.

SAMe reduces pain, fatigue and stiffness, improves serotonin synthesis which reduces pain perception, and supports liver detoxification. Patients on antidepressants or who have bipolar disorder should not take SAMe unless under strict supervision of their naturopath and doctor.

MSM reduces pain by preventing cartilage degeneration, reducing inflammation and boosting detoxification pathways.

Glucosamine reduces pain of joints in osteoarthritis.

Chondroitin reduces joint pain by drawing water into the cartilage matrix.

Homeopathy

Select one of the following remedies. Take two drops or pillules up to four times per day or until symptoms start to improve. Stop taking the remedy once symptoms resolve. If the symptoms return, take the remedy again until symptoms improve.

Rhus tox is used for stiffness and back pain, tearing pains and rheumatic pains. It is particularly useful when you feel better for movement or changing position, or when the weather is warm and dry. Rhus tox is also useful when the pain is worse at night time, when lying on your back or on your right hand side, during sleep, or when you get cold and wet.

Mag phos is good for muscular pain and back pain, especially if pain radiates to other parts of the body. It is indicated when the pain is accompanied by exhaustion, both physical and mental. When your pain is better for warm applications and pressure, and worse for cold weather or applications, mag phos will assist.

Arnica relieves general soreness, aching, bruises and the sensation of feeling bruised. It is well indicated when you feel better lying down or have your head down, and when you are worse from touch, motion, rest or cold.

Aurum is given for bone pain. It is particularly indicated when you feel depressed, when you desire being in the open air, and when you feel worse in cold weather and during the night.

Ars alb can relieve burning pains, especially when there is a burning thirst but you prefer to sip cold water frequently rather than drink large volumes at once. Ars Alb is very useful when there is also anxiety, restlessness or if you feel physically weak and chilly. The remedy is indicated when symptoms are worse when alone, around midnight, or are better for having company.

Hypericum is given for excessive nerve pains and injuries, especially of the fingers, toes and nails. It is very good for post-operative pain. Hypericum is specific for nerve sensations of tingling, burning and numbness. It is well indicated when the pain is accompanied by drowsiness, or when the pain is better for bending your head backward, or worse in cold, damp conditions. Hypericum is used when the pain is worse for touch.

Conium is specific for breast pain. It is also useful if you have difficulty walking, if you are trembling or have weakness while walking, or if you get painful stiffness in your legs. Conium is also used when there is poor memory. It has a positive effect on glands during cancer. If your pain feels better for fasting, or for being in a dark room, conium is indicated. It is also effective if your pain is better for letting your limbs hang down, and for applying pressure to the painful part. Conium is well indicated if your pain feels worse when you lie down, when you turn over in bed, when you get cold, or from physical or mental exertion.

Aromatherapy

Essential oils are complex substances that possess a vibrant quality and distinctive fragrance. They act on the body via inhalation, stimulating the olfactory nerve. A few drops of the following oils can be used in massage oil, added to a warm bath, or a vapouriser. They can be used individually or blended.

Lavender is used for pain, especially muscular spasm, cramping, low mood, headache and poor sleep.

Chamomile is effective for inflammation, headaches, nerve pain, muscle and back pain.

Clary sage relieves muscle spasm, aching and cramping.

Sweet marjoram relieves pain, stiffness, spasm, migraine and assists sleep.

Sandalwood is particularly good for pain associated with lymphatic congestion, making it well indicated for cancer.

The above oils can be combined with any of the citrus oils, which reduce tension and improve mood, including sweet orange, grapefruit, lemon, lime, tangerine and mandarin.

Anaemia

Anaemia can result from a range of causes, including a reduction in red cell production due to chemotherapy damage to bone marrow, blood loss during surgery, iron deficiency and folate or B12 deficiency. The cause of anaemia can be established with blood tests.

LOW RED CELL COUNT

Chemotherapy commonly causes suppression of bone marrow activity, responsible for creating a range of cells including red blood cells. Red blood cells are required to carry oxygen around the body, therefore decreased numbers lead to fatigue. Medical treatment may involve transfusions of packed blood cell products or erythropoietin, which increases production of red blood cells.

IRON DEFICIENCY ANAEMIA

A lack of dietary iron, poor digestion and absorption of iron, dysfunction of the liver, spleen and bone marrow, or loss of blood during surgery can all cause anaemia.

MEGALOBLASTIC ANAEMIA

Anaemia due to low folate or B12 levels is referred to as megaloblastic anaemia. This is usually due to poor levels in the diet. Low B12 levels may also be the result of pernicious anaemia, where the body cannot absorb B12 through the digestive tract.

Diet And Lifestyle

Iron is required for red blood cells to carry oxygen around the body. To maximize absorption of iron, adequate acidity is required in the stomach to break foods down; protein, B vitamins, choline and zinc are all required to make stomach acid. These can be found in a balanced diet including foods such as whole grains, green leafy vegetables, eggs, lentils, oats and the supplement lecithin. Absorption of iron is reduced by tea, coffee, antacids, vitamin E supplements, the food additive EDTA, aspirin, diarrhoea and laxative use.

In addition to iron, red blood cells require a range of other nutrients including protein, folate, copper and vitamins C, B6 and B12. These should be able to be obtained from a balanced diet.

Include quality protein sources such as beef and kangaroo, fish, eggs or chicken. Vegetarian protein sources include legumes and whole grains such as wholemeal bread, brown rice, nuts, seeds and oats. Protein powders can also be used. Many protein powders use whey protein that comes from dairy. Ask your naturopath for a soy or rice protein powder if you are sensitive to dairy.

Use organic meat, eggs, legumes and grains if available, as they are free from hormones, antibiotics and chemicals.

Herbal Medicine

A number of herbs are helpful in improving anaemia. They can be used individually or blended, and are taken as a liquid tincture, tablet or tea. Use under supervision of your naturopath.

Tincture doses are specific to each individual herb and can alter significantly depending on the strength and extraction process of the tincture.

Tablets are formulated at varying strengths, either alone or in combination with other herbs and nutrients.

Teas are made by diffusing the dried herb in boiled water, and are usually taken at three cups each day.

Dong quai is traditionally used as a blood tonic, improve red cell blood count.

Codonopsis is a blood tonic that improves haemoglobin production and red cell blood count.

Panax ginseng improves red blood cell count. It should not be used continuously for more than a couple of weeks without supervision. Be sure to consult your naturopath first to avoid interactions with any medications.

Nutrition

Specific nutrients can be used to support certain functions in the body. Although many of these are present in the diet, much higher levels of particular nutrients may be required.

Iron for iron-deficient anaemia. If a supplement is required, consider iron supplements in the form of ferrous fumarate, ferrous phosphate or ferrous gluconate as they are better absorbed than ferrous sulphate, which can also cause constipation.

Vitamin B12 for B12-deficient anaemia and in cases of suspected folate deficiency; folate deficiency signs can mask B12 deficiency. If B12 is deficient due to pernicious anaemia, injections or sublingual tablets are required.

Folate for folate-deficient anaemia. Higher doses than found in a multivitamin will be required.

Protein is required for building the globin component of haemoglobin, which carries iron around the body. Also required to make stomach acid to assist breakdown of iron for absorption.

Zinc is also required to build globin for haemoglobin, and for stomach acid production.

Vitamin C enhances iron absorption and reduces excretion of folate from the urinary system.

Vitamin B6 is required for haemoglobin synthesis, as well as energy production from protein and fats.

Copper is required if dietary measures are inadequate; a good quality multivitamin may maintain levels.

Fatigue

Fatigue is a symptom experienced by many people with cancer. This fatigue can originate from the cancer itself, cancer treatment (especially chemotherapy), the stress of dealing with cancer or as a result of bowel problems, insomnia, anaemia, lack of appetite or depression. It is important to realize that fatigue from cancer and its treatment is quite different to everyday fatigue, and may not respond as quickly to measures taken to improve it.

Diet And Lifestyle

A diet providing the full range of nutrients will best serve the body in recovering and restoring energy. A diet high in vegetables and fruit will maintain potassium levels, and this can help prevent muscle weakness and fatigue. Choose whole foods that have not been processed, such as whole grains, legumes, fresh vegetables and fruit, and nuts and seeds. Choose carbohydrates that are in their most natural state, such as brown rice, whole oats, grainy dark breads, legumes and root vegetables, and opt for proteins that are easy to digest.

Include good quality protein sources. Include lean red meat such as beef or kangaroo, as well as fish, eggs and chicken. Vegetarian protein sources include legumes and whole grains such as wholemeal bread, brown rice, nuts, seeds and oats. Protein powders can also be used. Many protein powders use whey protein that comes from dairy. Ask your naturopath for a soy or rice protein powder if you are sensitive to dairy.

Use organic meat, eggs, legumes and grains if available, as they are free from hormones, antibiotics and chemicals.

Good fats are an important source of energy, particularly when weight loss has been rapid and the body needs to store more fat. Look for good quality oils such as extra virgin olive oil, unsalted and unroasted nuts and avocado. Dairy can also be an important inclusion in the diet, however many people are intolerant to it, especially after chemotherapy. See your naturopath if you are concerned and would like to be tested for dairy intolerance or allergy.

Rest will give the body the greatest opportunity to recover from cancer treatments and also from dealing with the emotions of diagnosis and its impact on daily life and relationships. Avoid long sessions of activity and engagements, and ensure some quality rest time without television, computers or phones.

Gentle exercise is also recommended to maintain energy, muscle, bone density, cardiovascular health and mood. Choose an activity that you enjoy and engage at a level that is comfortable. Consider walking, bike riding, yoga, pilates and gentle weight training (under supervision). These can be done outside in the fresh air or using exercise equipment indoors, at home or at the gym.

Herbal Medicine

Due to the wide ranging causes of fatigue, many herbs have been found useful in restoring energy levels. Two groups of herbs that are often indicated in supporting cancer treatment are the adaptogens and thymoleptics. Adaptogens are traditionally understood to help the body adapt to change; physical, mental and emotional. Thymoleptics are known for their capacity to improve general mood. Use under supervision of your naturopath.

Tincture doses are specific to each individual herb and can alter significantly depending on the strength and extraction process of the tincture.

Tablets are formulated at varying strengths, either alone or in combination with other herbs and nutrients.

Teas are made by diffusing the dried herb in boiled water, and are usually taken at three cups each day.

Withania is an adaptogen that modifies the body's stress response, improves red blood cell production, supports the immune system, reduces inflammation and anxiety, supports mood, builds muscle mass and is protective to the liver and heart.

Panax ginseng is specifically used to support patients going through chemotherapy. Panax ginseng restores vitality, energy, cognitive function and mood, reduces inflammation and protects the liver and heart. It should not be used continuously for more than a couple of weeks without supervision. Be sure to consult your naturopath first to avoid interactions with any medications.

Siberian ginseng is known as an adaptogen that improves mood, supports immune function, modifies the body's stress response, reduces fatigue and raises vitality, builds muscle mass, improves mental and physical capacity, protects the liver and regulates blood sugar levels.

Cat's claw reduces fatigue, improves mood, supports immune and digestive function, and reduces oxidation and inflammation in the body.

Oats seed improves mood, relaxes nerves and regulates blood sugar levels.

Rhodiola is an adaptogen that improves mental clarity, mood and protects the liver while supporting its function.

Damiana is a mood enhancer and tonic to the nerves.

Nutrition

Specific nutrients can be used to support certain functions in the body. Although many of these are present in the diet, much higher levels of particular nutrients may be required.

B vitamins are very important for making energy from carbohydrates and fats in the diet. They are also important in supporting the nervous system's role in energy production, moderating the body's stress response and producing neurotransmitters required to maintain mood and sleep cycles.

Protein is essential for the body, and during chemotherapy it is particularly required to make new immune cells and rebuild muscle tissue. If dietary sources are not adequate, protein powders are an easy way to increase daily protein intake, and can be combined with fruit to add nutritional value and taste. Be aware that many protein powders use whey protein that comes from dairy. Ask your naturopath for a soy or rice protein powder if you are sensitive to dairy.

Iron is needed for red blood cells to carry oxygen around the body and to create enzymes required for energy production, hence good levels are required to combat fatigue.

Vitamin C is required for energy production, brain and nerve function, iron absorption, production of active folate, thyroid hormone and carnitine, all of which are necessary for good energy levels.

Zinc is needed for thyroid hormone conversion, uptake of glucose by cells for energy, to break down and metabolise food effectively and to build proteins required for brain function.

Homeopathy

Select one of the following remedies. Take two drops or pillules up to four times per day or until symptoms start to improve. Stop taking the remedy once symptoms resolve. If the symptoms return, take the remedy again until symptoms improve.

Kali phos is indicated for weakness and extreme physical and nervous exhaustion. It is useful when fatigue is caused by little exertion, stress, excessive worry, over excitement or working too much. Kali phos is particularly good for those who prefer to be alone, are irritable and sweat profusely.

Gels is effective when there is both physical and emotional weakness. It is particularly good when you have lost initiative, give up easily or doubt your ability to cope or perform well. Gels is typically used for excessive drowsiness and dizziness especially when accompanied by dull, persistent headaches, drooping eyelids or sore eyes. Feels worse for hot or humid weather.

Phos ac is used for fatigue and physical weakness when you are feeling particularly sensitive and easily overwhelmed by events around you. It is especially indicated if you feel indifferent, apathetic or have difficulty thinking clearly. Phos ac is effective when you have profuse perspiration, if you feel worse for the cold or become chilly easily, or if you feel particularly better for having rest or naps.

Ars alb is used for extreme fatigue accompanied by anxiety or restlessness. It is particularly indicated if you have a distinct fear of your cancer or of death. Fatigue and weakness may come and go quickly, especially after you exert yourself physically. Ars alb is also good if you are losing weight. If you are having burning sensations or pain, but feel chilly overall, then ars alb is likely to help your fatigue. It will also be helpful if your fatigue is worse when you are exposed to cold air or weather, or if it is worse at midnight.

Carbo veg is generally an excellent remedy for fatigue resulting from cancer, cancer treatments (including surgery), especially if you are also losing a lot of fluid through vomiting or diarrhoea. It is also effective if you have other digestive disturbances such as bloating and flatulence, especially if these are caused by eating fatty foods or if they improve after burping. When heat and humidity worsens your fatigue, Carbo veg is the best remedy to take.

Aromatherapy

Essential oils are complex substances that possess a vibrant quality and distinctive fragrance. They act on the body via inhalation, stimulating the olfactory nerve. A few drops of the following oils can be used in massage oil, added to a warm bath, or a vapouriser. They can be used individually or blended.

Rosemary enhances circulation to the brain, improving concentration.

Lavender is specific for alleviating nervous exhaustion.

Insomnia

Insomnia is difficulty falling or staying asleep. Many people with cancer experience it. Insomnia may be something you had experienced before your diagnosis of cancer, or the cancer itself can cause it. Cancer treatments can also contribute to poor sleep, as can the stress of dealing with cancer. Stress can increase the hormone cortisol and leave you too stimulated to sleep. It is important to realize that sleep is important for the immune system and the recovery from cancer and its treatment.

Diet And Lifestyle

Avoid foods that are stimulating as these tell your body it is time to be active, rather than rest. If you are unable to take these foods and drinks away completely, at least avoid them after midday. Stimulating foods include foods that are high in refined sugars, such as cakes, chocolate, biscuits, donuts and white bread. Alcohol, cigarettes and caffeine are also stimulants; avoid coffee, excessive black and green teas, and dark chocolate.

Include whole foods such as fruits, vegetables and protein. Proteins include lean red meat such as beef or kangaroo, as well as fish, eggs and chicken. Vegetarian protein sources include legumes and whole grains such as wholemeal bread, brown rice, nuts, seeds and oats. Protein powders can also be used. Many protein powders use whey protein that comes from dairy. Ask your naturopath for a soy or rice protein powder if you are sensitive to dairy.

Use organic meat, eggs, legumes and grains if available, as they are free from hormones, antibiotics and chemicals.

Our hormone levels play a large role in our sleeping habits. Having a routine helps to balance our hormone levels to improve sleep quality. Be in bed before 10pm and avoid bright white lights for at least thirty minutes before bed. This includes turning off televisions, computers and phones. Yellow light from a lamp does not affect our hormones, therefore it is fine to use just before bedtime. To relax at this time, read a book, have a bath or shower, or do a simple relaxation or meditation exercise.

Herbal Medicine

A number of herbs are helpful in reducing insomnia. A variety of herbs can be taken both during the day and night to relax the nervous system and enhance sleep quality. They can be used individually or blended, and are taken as a liquid tincture, tablet or tea. Use under supervision of your naturopath.

> *Tincture* doses are specific to each individual herb and can alter significantly depending on the strength and extraction process of the tincture.

> *Tablets* are formulated at varying strengths, either alone or in combination with other herbs and nutrients.

> *Teas* are made by diffusing the dried herb in boiled water, and are usually taken at three cups each day.

Valerian has been shown to have a positive effect on insomnia. It reduces anxiety, tones the nervous system and is gently sedating. Valerian also reduces muscle tension, restlessness and bloating. Best taken one to two hours before retiring, Valerian's effects increase after taking daily for at least two weeks.

Kava induces a more restful sleep, improves general mood and reduces anxiety without dampening alertness. It also reduces muscular spasm which can otherwise disrupt sleep.

Skullcap reduces insomnia by reducing nervous tension, agitation, restlessness, anxiety and muscle tension.

Chamomile has a relaxing action as well as a gentle sedating effect. It is useful when anxiety accompanies insomnia, when the mind is overactive and when the body is tired. It does this by regulating neurotransmitters that are over stimulated by stress.

Californian poppy has a gently sedating effect and reduces anxiety and pain.

Hops is particularly effective for insomnia associated with hot flushing. It enhances the body's natural sedating processes, reducing agitation, excitability and nervous exhaustion. Hops is also effective for nerve pain, headaches and nervous tension in the gut. A bath with hops added to the warm water improves sleep quality when repeated each evening.

Passionflower provides a gentle sedative action and reduces restlessness, anxiety, muscle spasm and pain. Passionflower is especially good for broken sleep and insomnia caused by jet lag or shift work. It is best taken just before bed to prevent waking during the night. Use of passionflower should be avoided if there is a tendency to migraines, or if taking beta blocker blood pressure medication.

Ziziphus is a sedating herb that is particularly useful if sweating during the night contributes to poor sleep quality.

Nutrition

Specific nutrients can be used to support certain functions in the body. Although many of these are present in the diet, much higher levels of particular nutrients may be required.

Magnesium is a common deficiency in people with insomnia. It is required for the production of neurotransmitters that regulate mood, for nerve conduction, relaxation of muscles and production of energy at the cellular level. Signs of magnesium deficiency include muscle twitches and cramps, quivering tongue and eye twitching. Magnesium levels are depleted by stress; physical, mental and emotional.

B vitamins support the nervous system and improve sleep patterns.

Calcium is required for the nervous system, production of neurotransmitters, and is involved in maintaining healthy sleep cycles.

Homeopathy

Select one of the following remedies. Take two drops or pillules up to four times per day or until symptoms start to improve. Stop taking the remedy once symptoms resolve. If the symptoms return, take the remedy again until symptoms improve.

Nux Vom is used when you can get to sleep fine, but you wake up during the night, especially around 3am, and then feel terrible in the morning. It is particularly indicated if you are stressed and irritable. Nux vom is well indicated if you have constipation, if you are oversensitive, or if your insomnia is due to overindulging in stimulants.

Coffea helps insomnia that is accompanied by an overactive mind, too much caffeine intake, great nervous agitation and restlessness or extreme nervous excitability. It is used for feeling overstimulated from too much excitement or sudden emotions. It is also used when pain tolerance is very low and the pain drives you to the point of despair.

Pulsatilla is effective for insomnia when you can't sleep on your own, when your sleep pattern is changeable and when you are emotionally sensitive. It is also good if you are sweating excessively but are rarely thirsty. Pulsatilla is indicated if you generally feel better from having the window open, having company, having a good cry or regularly push the bed covers off during the night. It is also useful if your sleep is worse when lying on your left side.

Ars alb is helpful when insomnia is worse around midnight, or if you feel anxiety or even panicky. If you are greatly fatigued but restless, and wake unrefreshed, ars alb is indicated. Dreaming especially of storms, fires or darkness are characteristics of this remedy. There may also be a sensation of a burning under the skin.

Bell is for restlessness and being woken by anxious and vivid nightmares. Jerking during sleep, feeling drowsy and yawning in evening also indicate this remedy. Bell is useful if you have a pounding sensation in the head, if you can hear blood pulsating in the head, or if you wake with a headache.

Nat mur is indicated if you can't sleep when someone else is in the bed, or if you have a fear of intruders. If you especially desire to be alone, dwell on past disappointments, or feel bitter, this remedy is indicated. Nat mur is also used when there is sleeplessness from grief (especially if you don't talk about the grief), feel angry or sleep walk. It is well indicated if you generally feel worse when consoled.

Sulphur is for insomnia due to irritability, getting too hot in bed, or when you also have itchy or burning soles of the feet. If you feel better for uncovering your feet, have great thirst, or if you also have diarrhoea that drives you out of bed, Sulphur is a useful remedy.

Silica is indicated for insomnia when you are anxious, sensitive, and are resistant to change. If you can't sleep because your feet are cold, or you are very thirsty, have a headache or have numb sensations in the body, Silica may be the correct remedy. It is used in those who feel worse when they are cold, after mental exhaustion or when they feel worse after rest, or for being consoled.

Bach Flower Essences

These may be combined or used individually. Take four drops under the tongue four times a day.

Aspen is for unexplained fears and worries, and when nervous or anxious.

White chestnut for an overactive mind, unwanted thoughts, preoccupations and worries.

Impatiens is for impatience and irritation.

Aromatherapy

Essential oils are complex substances that possess a vibrant quality and distinctive fragrance. They act on the body via inhalation, stimulating the olfactory nerve. A few drops of the following oils can be used in massage oil, added to a warm bath, or a vapouriser. They can be used individually or blended.

Lavender improves sleep quality. Its aroma is specific for nervous tension, and is calming and soothing with gentle sedative effects. It has been shown to reduce hyperactivity caused by caffeine. Lavender inhalation also improves mood and reduces anxiety.

Chamomile has a relaxing action as well as a gentle sedating effect. It is useful when anxiety accompanies insomnia or when the mind keeps going even though the body is tired. Chamomile reduces the levels of neurotransmitters that are produced during stress.

Depression

Depression can be a part of the cancer journey and may begin after the shock of cancer diagnosis. The fatigue of the cancer itself as well as the medical treatment can also contribute to low mood. Spending a lot of time indoors when ill can reduce sun exposure and may lead to low vitamin D levels. This in itself can cause low mood, also known as Seasonal Affective Disorder. Regardless of the cause, feelings of sadness and grief are a normal part of life, however it is important to be aware if they become more permanent than transient.

In addition to beneficial naturopathic remedies, counselling can be helpful and effective in addressing depression.

Diet And Lifestyle

Avoid refined foods and foods that are high in sugar such as cakes, biscuits, donuts and white bread. These foods cause blood sugar fluctuations, leading to low mood when blood sugar levels plummet.

Include whole foods such as fruits, vegetables and protein. Proteins include lean red meat such as beef or kangaroo, as well as fish, eggs and chicken. Vegetarian protein sources include legumes and whole grains such as wholemeal bread, brown rice, nuts, seeds and oats. Protein powders can also be used. Many protein powders use whey protein that comes from dairy. Ask your naturopath for a soy or rice protein powder if you are sensitive to dairy.

Use organic meat, eggs, legumes and grains if available, as they are free from hormones, antibiotics and chemicals.

Good fats (omega 3) are important for brain function as our brains are made mostly of fat. Look for oily fish such as salmon, tuna, mackerel, sardines, herring, swordfish, rainbow trout, oysters and mussels. Good quality fats also come from coconut oil, extra virgin olive oil, nuts, seeds and avocado.

Exercise is as important for mood as it is for cardiovascular function. Include regular movement (walking, stretching, yoga) that is applicable to your health level.

Sensible sun exposure is also important for activating vitamin D in the body. Avoid being out in the sun during the hottest part of the day, and when you do go out, only expose your skin for short periods of time.

Herbal Medicine

A number of herbs are helpful in improving depression. A variety of herbs can be taken both during the day and night to relax the nervous system and enhance mood. They can be used individually or blended, and are taken as a liquid tincture, tablet or tea. Use under supervision of your naturopath. If you are currently taking antidepressants, consult your doctor before making any changes to your medication.

> **Tincture** doses are specific to each individual herb and can alter significantly depending on the strength and extraction process of the tincture.

> **Tablets** are formulated at varying strengths, either alone or in combination with other herbs and nutrients.

> **Teas** are made by diffusing the dried herb in boiled water, and are usually taken at three cups each day.

St John's Wort has been shown to successfully treat mild to moderate depression. It has many drug interactions so should only be taken under the supervision of a qualified naturopath, particularly if taking medications. St John's Wort also acts on the nervous system to reduce anxiety, thereby improving general mood and sleep.

Rhodiola has been shown to be as effective as anti depressants in treating mild to moderate depression.

Damiana has traditionally been used as a general tonic to enhance mood and increase libido. It is especially good for men.

Rosemary is used if low mood is characterized by physical exhaustion, mental fatigue and poor memory.

Ginkgo reduces depression and anxiety by assisting production of mood regulating neurotransmitters and their receptors, improving circulation to the brain and protecting nerve pathways.

Oats have traditionally been used for low mood, fatigue and periods of convalescence.

Nutrition

Specific nutrients can be used to support certain functions in the body. Although many of these are present in the diet, much higher levels of particular nutrients may be required.

A deficiency of any nutrient can affect brain function and contribute to depression. The following nutrients are the most common deficiencies seen with low mood.

B vitamins support nerve and immune function. They are required for the body to produce energy and play a role in many biochemical reactions. Look for good levels of B6, B12 and folate in supplements.

Magnesium is a common deficiency in depression. It is required for the production of neurotransmitters that regulate mood, as well as nerve conduction, relaxation of muscles and production of energy at the cellular level. Signs of magnesium deficiency include muscle twitches and cramps, quivering tongue and eye twitches. Magnesium levels are depleted by stress; physical, mental and emotional.

Vitamin C is involved in the production of neurotransmitters that regulate mood. Higher levels of vitamin C have been correlated with increased cancer survival.

Zinc is required for optimal neurological function and deficiency of the mineral is associated with depression.

Omega 3 deficiency compromises the nervous system's capacity to stimulate mood. As well as eating omega 3 foods, an omega 3 supplement such as fish oil can eliminate deficiency and optimize nervous system function and mood. See your naturopath to ensure you choose a fish oil that is protected from oxidation during processing and storage, and has sufficient levels of EPA and DHA for a therapeutic effect.

Homeopathy

Select one of the following remedies. Take two drops or pillules up to four times per day or until symptoms start to improve. Stop taking the remedy once symptoms resolve. If the symptoms return, take the remedy again until symptoms improve.

Aurum is indicated if you are in despair, feel dissatisfaction, experience low self esteem, have feelings of hopelessness, loathe life or cannot find joy in any activities or relationships. Aurum is the remedy for you if you often hide depression so others are unaware of it. You may be overly critical of yourself and others, condemn yourself, and are quarrelsome, irritable and easily angered. Aurum is also used when you feel you have lost the affection of friends. Characteristically, those who benefit from Aurum desire open air, feel worse in the cold weather, and worse overnight. It is especially useful in cases of bone cancer.

Ignatia is for depression associated with grief and fears. There may also be significant mood swings, self-reproach, shame and silent grief. It is characteristically indicated for romantics, idealists and those with a strong sense of responsibility. You may feel irritability that is worse for consolation and be very sensitive to touch, cigarette smoke and coffee.

Pulsatilla is for irritability, changeability, feeling timid and weeping often, especially when speaking about depression. There can be a tendency to self-pitying. This remedy is indicated if you crave open air, feel better for sympathy and cold food and drinks, and feel worse in a warm stuffy room.

Sepia is especially effective in women. It is used when you feel apathy towards loved ones, are averse to company and cut yourself off from others even though you dread being alone. Changeable emotions, being disagreeable, feeling chilly and feeling better for vigorous exercise are characteristics of someone who requires Sepia.

Nat mur is for you if you are very sensitive to rejection and criticism, brood over old insults, feel bleak and cheerless and are worse for being consoled. It is indicated for more consistent and profound depression than Ignatia. Depression that benefits from nat mur is often a development from an emotional vulnerability that becomes melancholic. As the depression worsens you do nothing to try and relieve it. People needing nat mur often feel worse for sunlight and heat, but better for open air and being flexible with meal times.

Phos ac is for apathy, indifference, resignation, dullness, passive behaviour, feeling overwhelmed, having difficulty putting words or thoughts together and feeling listless and weak. It is well indicated when there is loss of appetite and night sweats. If you feel worse after sleep, overwork, study or grief, or are feeling burn out generally, Phos ac is an effective remedy.

Bach Flower Essences

Gorse is used for utter despondency and hopelessness.

Gentian is for when you feel discouraged, hesitant and despondent.

Mustard is for when you are experiencing unexplained deep gloom that comes and goes without an apparent reason.

Olive is for feeling exhausted in body and mind.

Wild rose is for when you feel apathetic and make little effort to improve situations.

Aromatherapy

Essential oils are complex substances that possess a vibrant quality and distinctive fragrance. They act on the body via inhalation, stimulating the olfactory nerve. A few drops of the following oils can be used in massage oil, added to a warm bath, or a vapouriser. They can be used individually or blended.

Neroli is uplifting and nourishing.

Cardomom is used for apathy, lethargy and emotional exhaustion. It is uplifting without overstimulating.

Geranium is used to relieve nervousness, uneasiness and depression.

Bergamot refreshes and relaxes the nerves.

Rosemary is relaxing, brings clarity and perspective.

Chamomile is used when depression is moody, irritable and dissatisfied.

Rose is used for a lack of enthusiasm, to inspire and rebalance.

Lemon can be helpful for depressed moods due to its refreshing, sharp aspects.

Lavender improves mood and sleep quality. It reduces nervous tension, and is calming and soothing with gentle sedative effects.

Anxiety

Although anxiety is within the normal spectrum of emotional experience, at times our nervous system can become so overactive that we find ourselves in a constant state of heightened worry or concern. When experiencing such ongoing anxiety, the body's mood regulators, neurotransmitters, become dysregulated and continuously stimulate the stress response. The body is then in an ongoing state of stress which quickly depletes energy resources and compromises immune function.

Diet And Lifestyle

To reduce the overactivity of the nervous system, stimulants need to be avoided as much as possible. Stimulants commonly disrupt sleep patterns, reducing regenerative sleep that the body requires when coping with anxiety. Stimulants include refined sugars, alcohol, cigarettes and caffeine. Reduce your intake of sugars by avoiding table sugar, chocolate, lollies and refined carbohydrates such as white bread and pasta; refined carbohydrates are quickly broken down into sugars by the body. Although alcohol can help reduce anxiety in the short term, it will contribute to wiping out energy levels and is likely to lead to more long term issues with both anxiety and depression. Caffeine is also a stimulant and causes hyperactivity. It increases our blood pressure and our alertness. Avoid caffeinated drinks; these include cola, energy drinks and coffee. Smaller amounts of caffeine are also found in black and green teas, and dark chocolate.

The nervous system requires significant amounts of B vitamins and magnesium, therefore when it is overactive with anxiety, we become depleted in these nutrients. Increase your food sources of B vitamins and magnesium by eating oats, brown rice and green leafy vegetables such as broccoli, spinach, cauliflower, silver beet and brussel sprouts.

Breathing exercises are one of the most powerful methods to reduce anxiety. Spend five minutes a day focusing on your breath. Whenever you catch yourself in an anxious state, take some deeper breaths and when you can, take a few minutes to observe your breath moving in and out of the body.

Relaxation activities are invaluable when experiencing anxiety. Every day do something you find relaxing, such as yoga, having a relaxation massage or bath, taking a class in qi gong or meditation, or going for a walk at the beach or through parkland.

Identify the people around you that are most helpful to talk to about your anxiety. Be aware if talking about your anxiety makes it worse. If this is the case, limit the number of people you choose to discuss your anxiety with, and how much time you spend talking about it. Focusing on the positives of how you are coping with the anxiety is more helpful than looking at the negative effects of being anxious. Professional psychological support is highly recommended.

Herbal Medicine

A number of herbs are helpful in reducing anxiety. A variety of herbs can be taken both during the day and night. They can be used individually or blended, and are taken as a liquid tincture, tablet or tea. Use under supervision of your naturopath.

> **Tincture** doses are specific to each individual herb and can alter significantly depending on the strength and extraction process of the tincture.

> **Tablets** are formulated at varying strengths, either alone or in combination with other herbs and nutrients.

Teas are made by diffusing the dried herb in boiled water, and are usually taken at three cups each day.

Kava acts on the nervous system to reduce anxiety and relax muscles, and improves pain, general mood and sleep.

St John's Wort has anti-anxiety effects. It is useful when there is also mild to moderate depression or ongoing stress. As it has many interactions with medications it is important to use St John's Wort under the supervision of a qualified naturopath.

Lavender helps with relaxation. It has been shown to reduce hyperactivity caused by caffeine. Lavender inhalation improves mood and reduces anxiety.

Chamomile reduces levels of neurotransmitters that are produced during stress. It contains relaxation and anti-anxiety properties. Chamomile is especially useful if anxiety accompanies poor sleep.

Passion flower has an anti-anxiety action. At high doses it provides a sedative action. It can be taken before bed to prevent waking during the night.

Valerian has been shown to reduce anxiety and psychological stress. It also has a positive effect on insomnia in numerous studies. It is best taken one to two hours before retiring.

Withania reduces anxiety, modulates the stress response and enhances memory. Through its antioxidant and anti-inflammatory properties it has been shown to have anticancer activity.

Nutrition

Specific nutrients can be used to support certain functions in the body. Although many of these are present in the diet, much higher levels of particular nutrients may be required.

B vitamins are used by the body to build neurotransmitters that stabilize mood. B vitamins are also needed by the adrenal glands to enable the body to deal with high levels of ongoing stress. B vitamins improve energy levels, enhance sleep quality and reduce fatigue. They are quickly depleted by anxiety and stress.

Magnesium is required by the adrenal glands to respond to stress. It is also needed to relax muscle contractions, calm the nervous system and produce energy. It is quickly depleted by anxiety and stress; physical, mental and emotional.

L-Glutamine is required for the production of neurotransmitters involved in relaxing the nervous system. It is particularly useful when anxiety is associated with gut disturbances.

Homeopathy

Select one of the following remedies. Take two drops or pillules up to four times per day or until symptoms start to improve. Stop taking the remedy once symptoms resolve. If the symptoms return, take the remedy again until symptoms improve.

Aconite is given for anxiety with great fear, especially of death, or worry from shock. If you have panic, excitability, or claustrophobia, aconite is indicated. It is also used to reduce pain sensitivity.

Ars alb is for anxiety with fear, guilt, resentment, uncertainty, worry, restlessness and physical weakness. It is also for anxiety that is worse when alone and around midnight. If you have a tendency to blame others, ars alb is the remedy. If you are complaining, critical or also depressed, but feel better for company, this remedy is indicated. Ars alb is also helpful if you have a burning thirst for sips of cold water, or you generally feel extremely chilly.

Calc carb is for anxiety with fatigue, dread and claustrophobia. It differentiated from aconite because the anxiety comes with sweet cravings. You may feel so chilly it is difficult to stay warm. Calc carb is also used if you have a specific fear of heights.

Kali phos is for when anxiety leads to exhaustion or illness. There may also be insomnia, oversensitivity, agitation, poor concentration or poor adaptability to stress. You have a desire to talk about your problems and a fear of not being able to cope.

Coffea is for anxiety with hypersensitivity to noise and an overactive mind. If you have insomnia due to too much caffeine, great nervous agitation and restlessness, or extreme nervous excitability, coffea is indicated. It is also used when pain is driving you to despair, especially after sudden emotions.

Bell is indicated for anxiety that rises suddenly, with restlessness, overexcitement or being woken by anxious and vivid nightmares. If you twitch or jerk during sleep and are drowsy and yawning in evening, Bell is indicated. This remedy is useful if you wake with a headache, especially if it is pounding headache, or you can hear blood pulsing in your head. Bell is used if the face is red, hot and flushed, eyes are glaring, or the mouth and throat are dry but with no thirst.

Bach Flower Essences

Aspen is for unexplained fears and worries, with feelings of nervousness and anxiety.

White chestnut is for an overactive mind, with unwanted thoughts, preoccupations and worries. It is used when your mind won't slow down and is constantly busy with thought.

Impatiens is for feelings of impatience and irritation.

Star of Bethlehem is for the effects of shock, grief or fright, especially indicated for the shock of a diagnosis.

Cherry plum is for when you feel fearful of losing control of your behaviour.

Rock rose is used for feelings of helplessness, terror or feeling frozen in fear.

Clematis is for daydreaming and a general lack of interest in what is happening in the present.

Rescue remedy is a combination of five Bach Flower essences that are specific for demanding or stressful situations.

Aromatherapy

Essential oils are complex substances that possess a vibrant quality and distinctive fragrance. They act on the body via inhalation, stimulating the olfactory nerve. A few drops of the following oils can be used in massage oil, added to a warm bath, or a vapouriser. They can be used individually or blended.

Geranium is used to relieve nervousness, uneasiness and depression.

Bergamot refreshes and relaxes the nerves.

Rosemary is relaxing, brings clarity and perspective.

Chamomile is used when there is depression with moodiness, irritability and dissatisfaction.

Lavender improves mood and sleep quality. It reduces nervous tension, and is calming and soothing with gentle sedative effects.

Stress

Stress produces a biological response in our bodies. There are three phases of the stress response, and each may play a role in cancer.

The first phase of stress is "fight or flight", where our bodies release adrenalin and the hormone cortisol in order to raise our physiological capacity to deal with the immediate stress.

After the stressful event is over, our adrenalin and cortisol levels return to normal. Under prolonged stress however, the body doesn't have a chance to return to normal, and we enter the second phase of the stress response called the "resistance" phase. Cortisol levels remain high, and put increased demands on our heart, blood vessels, adrenal glands and immune system. The body is in a constant state of stress response and doesn't get the rest it needs to recover. If the body is in resistance phase during cancer, it has less capacity to fight the cancer and cope with chemotherapy and radiotherapy treatments.

If the body remains in the "resistance" phase for months or years, the body may eventually lose its capacity to produce enough cortisol to give us the energy we need for daily living, and we enter the third phase known as "adrenal fatigue." Dealing with cancer while adrenally fatigued becomes even more challenging, and supporting the adrenal glands becomes a priority.

Recognizing stress in yourself is not always easy. You may notice physical signs of stress, which can include insomnia, depression, fatigue, headache, upset stomach, digestive problems and irritability. Diarrhoea is particularly common when people are stressed, anxious or nervous; the brain chemical that increases when we are stressed acts directly on the digestive tract and this can increase bowel activity.

The key to dealing with stress effectively is to improve the capacity to adapt. We can do this through eating well, exercising, taking supplements that support our physiological stress response and improving our mental and emotional resistance to stress.

Diet And Lifestyle

Stimulants increase our stress response and should be avoided as much as possible. These include sugars and caffeine. Reduce your intake of sugars by avoiding sugar, chocolate, lollies and refined carbohydrates such as white bread and pasta; refined carbohydrates are quickly broken down into sugars by the body.

Include foods rich in B vitamins and magnesium as we use high levels of these nutrients when we are stressed. Quality food sources include oats, brown rice and green leafy vegetables such as broccoli, spinach, cauliflower, silver beet and brussel sprouts.

When under stress, the body prioritizes its blood supply and energy to the muscles and brain. To improve digestion, sit down and relax before you start eating. Planning meals ahead of time will help take the stress out of eating, and allows choice of healthier meals rather than just eating what is left in the cupboard.

Reduce alcohol intake and stimulants such as coffee and cigarettes. These put the body under a lot of pressure, particularly the liver which is required to clear out the by products of the body's stress response. Stimulants commonly disrupt sleep patterns, reducing regenerative sleep that the body requires from being caught up in the stress response.

It is important to identify any food allergies, as allergic responses cause a stress response in the body, leading to high cortisol levels. Your naturopath can test you for specific food allergies.

One of the most powerful methods to reduce stress and increase energy is to focus on your breath and take some deeper breaths. If breathing is deep, it will involve your diaphragm; you will be able to observe your abdomen moving in and out. If breathing is shallow, it may only involve your chest; when this happens your shoulders and rib cage are more likely to be moving up and down. Spend at least five minutes a day focusing on your breath.

Also spend some time each day doing an activity you find relaxing. Qi gong, yoga and meditation are highly beneficial in reducing the stress response. Daily activities can also be relaxing, such as reading, taking a warm bath, going for a walk in a natural environment or having a massage.

Bringing a more positive outlook to your relationships will help keep things in perspective and increase your appreciation for the support you already have. Remember that those closest to you may also be feeling stressed at this time. Positive communication encourages positive responses back to you.

Psychological support is highly recommended to optimize your capacity to deal with the mental and emotional impact of cancer, as well as improving your capacity to heal and recover.

Herbal Medicine

A number of herbs are helpful in reducing stress. A variety of herbs can be taken both during the day and night to relax the nervous system. They can be used individually or blended, and are taken as a liquid tincture, tablet or tea. Use under supervision of your naturopath.

> *Tincture* doses are specific to each individual herb and can alter significantly depending on the strength and extraction process of the tincture.

Tablets are formulated at varying strengths, either alone or in combination with other herbs and nutrients.

Teas are made by diffusing the dried herb in boiled water, and are usually taken at three cups each day.

Withania modulates the stress response as well as enhancing memory. Through its antioxidant and anti-inflammatory properties it has been shown to have an anticancer action.

Licorice is used for long term stress when the adrenal glands are under functioning. It reduces breakdown of the stress hormone cortisol, extending its capacity to deal with stress. For this reason, it should be avoided if cortisol levels are too high. See your naturopath to assess your hormone levels and decide if licorice will benefit your particular type of stress. Licorice is not recommended for long term use or for those with high blood pressure or on some heart medications.

Rehmannia also restores the adrenal glands and helps the body adapt to stress. It also has potent anti-inflammatory properties, modulates the immune system and enhances kidney function.

Siberian ginseng increases resistance to stress, normalizing the body's response during stressful periods.

Kava acts on the nervous system to reduce anxiety and relax muscles. It improves pain, general mood and sleep.

St John's Wort has anti-anxiety effects. It is useful when mild to moderate depression is accompanying ongoing stress. As it has many interactions with medications, St John's Wort must be used under the supervision of a qualified naturopath.

Lavender helps with relaxation. It has been shown to reduce hyperactivity caused by caffeine. Lavender inhalation improves mood and reduces anxiety.

Chamomile reduces levels of neurotransmitters that are produced during stress. It contains relaxation and anti-anxiety properties.

Passion flower has an anti-anxiety action. At high doses it provides a sedative action. It can be taken before bed to prevent waking during the night.

Valerian has been shown to reduce anxiety and psychological stress. It also has a positive effect on insomnia in numerous studies. It is best taken one to two hours before retiring.

Panax ginseng is used for stress and cancer. It should not be used continuously for more than a couple of weeks. Be sure to consult your naturopath first to avoid interactions with any medications.

Nutrition

Specific nutrients can be used to support certain functions in the body. Although many of these are present in the diet, much higher levels of particular nutrients may be required.

B vitamins are used by the body to build neurotransmitters that help to stabilize mood. They are also needed by the adrenal glands to enable the body to deal with high levels of ongoing stress. B vitamins improve energy levels, enhance sleep quality and reduce fatigue. They are quickly depleted by anxiety and stress.

Magnesium is required by the adrenal glands to respond to stress. It is also needed to relax muscle contractions, calm the nervous system and produce energy. It is quickly depleted by anxiety and stress; physical, mental and emotional.

Vitamin C is also required for optimal adrenal function in the stress response and lowers the stress hormone cortisol during the stress response. It is involved in neurotransmitter synthesis and is required to make energy.

Zinc is needed by the adrenal glands during the stress response.

L-Glutamine is required for the production of neurotransmitters involved in relaxing the nervous system. It is particularly useful when anxiety is associated with gut disturbances.

Homeopathy

Select one of the following remedies. Take two drops or pillules up to four times per day or until symptoms start to improve. Stop taking the remedy once symptoms resolve. If the symptoms return, take the remedy again until symptoms improve.

Aconite is for stress with great fear, especially of death, or worry from shock. Anxiety, panic, excitability and claustrophobia are all signs that aconite is the correct remedy. Increased sensitivity to pain, fear and being worse from shock are all indicators for aconite.

Ars alb is indicated for fear, guilt, resentment, uncertainty, worry, restlessness and physical weakness. It is used if you have stress with anxiety that is worse when alone and around midnight. Ars alb is often used when there is a burning thirst for sips of cold water and you feel extremely chilly.

Aurum is indicated when you feel hopeless, despondent, betrayed, guilty, lonely or ashamed. It is also used when you feel like a failure, are experiencing loss, or if you are angry but have difficulty expressing it.

Calc carb is given for illness caused by stress, fatigue, anxiety or dread. It is particularly useful if you also have claustrophobia, sweet cravings or get so chilly you cannot get warm. Calc carb is specific for a fear of heights.

Gels is used for stress that causes weakness, trembling, chills, perspiration, diarrhoea, headaches and mental dullness. If you have anticipatory anxiety or a specific fear of crowds, or of falling, gels is indicated.

Ignatia is for stress caused by grief and loss, disappointment, criticism or loneliness.

Kali phos is for stress that leads to exhaustion or illness. If you have stress with insomnia, oversensitivity, agitated anxiety, poor concentration or poor adaptability to stress, then kali phos is useful. It is also indicated if you have a desire to talk about your problems, or have a fear of not being able to cope.

Coffea is for stress with a high sensitivity to noise and an overactive mind. If your insomnia is due to too much caffeine or if you are particularly nervous, agitated and restless, then coffea is indicated. It is a remedy for extreme nervous excitability and intolerance of pain that can drive you to despair. Coffea is also for insomnia after sudden emotions.

Bell is for stress that comes on suddenly, with restlessness and overexcitement. If you are woken by anxious and vivid nightmares, or twitch or jerk during sleep, bell is the correct remedy. It is also used for drowsiness and yawning in the evening, pounding in the head, hearing blood pulsing in head and if you wake with a headache. Bell is typically used when you have a red face, get hot and flushed easily, when your eyes are glaring or when your mouth and throat are dry but you are not thirsty.

Bach Flower Essences

Aspen is for unexplained fears and worries, when feeling nervous and anxious.

White chestnut is for having an overactive mind. If you have unwanted thoughts, preoccupations and worries, then white chestnut is indicated.

Impatiens is indicated if you feel impatient and irritated.

Star of Bethlehem is for the effects of shock, grief or fright. It is especially indicated for the shock of a diagnosis.

Cherry plum is indicated when you are fearful of losing control of your behaviour.

Rock rose is used if you have feelings of terror, helplessness of feel frozen in fear.

Clematis is for daydreaming and having a general lack of interest in what is happening.

Rescue remedy is a combination of five Bach Flower essences that are specific for demanding or stressful situations.

Aromatherapy

Essential oils are complex substances that possess a vibrant quality and distinctive fragrance. They act on the body via inhalation, stimulating the olfactory nerve. A few drops of the following oils can be used in massage oil, added to a warm bath, or a vapouriser. They can be used individually or blended.

Geranium is used to relieve nervousness, uneasiness and depression.

Bergamot refreshes and relaxes the nerves.

Rosemary is relaxing, brings clarity and perspective.

Chamomile is used when there is depression with moodiness, irritability and dissatisfaction.

Lavender improves mood and sleep quality. It reduces irritability, nervous tension, and is calming and soothing with gentle sedative effects.

Psychology, Cancer and Recovery

Campbell Thompson
Psychologist. Bachelor Science (Honours), Masters Degree Psychology

Speaking with a psychologist can be of great help to people with cancer in a number of ways. It can help to lessen the emotional distress of dealing with diagnosis, symptoms, treatment and its side effects, as well as helping families and friends to communicate about what is important and improve the quality of daily interactions and life in general. In terms of healing and recovery, psychological support can also promote immune function and optimize the body's capacity to recover from cancer and its treatments.

More than 50% of Australians in treatment for cancer have used some form of psychological therapy. Given the significance of the changes to our way of life that come with a cancer diagnosis, expectations are often high; 25% of patients expect the psychological therapy to cure cancer, and 75-100% expect it to assist traditional therapy. Although these expectations are high, almost 100% of patients indicated their satisfaction with therapy, recommending psychology to other patients and stating they would use these therapies again. The Ontario Cancer Institute recently ran a research study with a group of patients with seemingly incurable cancer. They concluded that those who worked the hardest at transforming themselves psychologically had the best survival rates. When we take an active role in our own well-being, aim to create an environment where the body can heal itself, work with our bodies and not against them, then we give our bodies the best chance they have of recovering from illness. These measures also allow us to enjoy more of the meaningful and important moments that make up our day to day lives.

PSYCHOLOGY AND HEALING

Every emotion has a physiological impact on the body, especially when it is sustained over time. Emotions, both pleasant and unpleasant, are a normal and healthy part of the ebb and flow of our experience. But when we hold onto these emotions, or when they turn into persistent anxiety or dread, they can compromise the immune system and our physical health.

When faced with a challenge such as a cancer diagnosis, none of these "gut reactions" are bad or wrong. But they do not need to define our experience going forward. Fighting is a gut instinct, and is sometimes encouraged when faced with a cancer, but "fighting" is most effective when it does not involve anger, fear or anxiety. Speaking with a psychologist can teach us to manage these emotions and reduce their impact on our physical health.

PSYCHOLOGY AND PAIN

Significant or chronic pain is an emotional experience as much as a physical one. It can affect all aspects of your life, including relationships with loved ones. People with chronic pain regularly describe how distress, anger, depression and anxiety result from their pain when it's left unchecked.

Thinking about pain and actively dreading it actually induces even higher levels of pain. Initially, pain is experienced when part of the body is injured or hurt, sending a pain signal to the brain and this creates what we feel as pain. When this pathway is repeated often enough, the brain can also actively tune in to these pain signals from a particular part of the body, and become more sensitive to pain from these areas. Habits and expectations of pain can increase this "sensitization," and in this state of "pain alertness" even a small pain signal can result in an intense pain experience. Emotional states like anxiety and fear also increase pain sensitization. Psychotherapy techniques can be used to minimize this type of pain sensitivity, radically reduce our experience of pain and give us the capacity to focus our energy and attention on what we value.

MENTAL IMAGERY IN HEALING AND REHABILITATION

Mental Imagery involves creating rich internal images using visualization, sense of hearing, touch and even smell, while in a state of deep relaxation. By creating rich internal images of the body healing itself and overcoming illness in a natural way, an environment for optimal healing is created.

Chronic illness can lead people to resent their bodies or feel let down by them. It is possible to harbour anger, frustration and even hate, or experience persistent grief regarding the loss of health or function of the body in some way. Intense emotions can block recovery, and sleep, rest and relaxation become compromised. Practicing mental imagery regularly allows anger and resentment to give way to peace, acceptance, warmth and self-compassion. This allows recovery and quality of life to be enhanced.

Other types of mental imagery involve the creation of a place of retreat or an internal sanctuary. When going through painful treatment and side effects, it is possible for the mind to take you to a beautiful beach in the South Pacific, hearing the sea and feeling the sun and warm breeze on your skin. Experiences like these can help in dealing with pain, but they also help us reconnect to the beauty and peace that still exists in the world despite the unpleasant experience that may be dominating our thinking and awareness at a given time.

A recent scientific review of 329 studies showed that mental imagery reduced pain in 86% of studies on cancer patients, and relaxation training and imagery were supported as showing positive effects on not just quality of life, but also immune and survival outcomes.

MINDFULNESS

Mindfulness involves bringing attention to your present moment experience in an open, caring and non-judging way. When we see our thoughts, emotions and sensations rise and fall without getting caught up in them, we can avoid the fallout of holding stress, fear and anxiety in our bodies. Aside from reducing enjoyment of our lives, these emotions can also reduce the effectiveness of our immune, digestive and reproductive systems. By practicing mindfulness, and choosing to let go of anxious preoccupations, we can create an environment in which our bodies can more easily heal themselves, and make best use of the medical care we are already receiving.

The psychologist Elana Rosenbaum writes about her experiences with mindfulness and cancer in the book *Here for Now: Living Well With Cancer Through Mindfulness*. She describes her experience with mindfulness meditation when she contracted pneumonia after stem-cell treatment for an aggressive lymphoma:

> *My ability to quiet the mind, and just be there breath by breath, without heightening or contracting in response to what was happening, allowed me to breathe better. Without mindfulness during that period, I actually believe I would have died.*

She goes on to describe how, even through the hardest times, in opening up her awareness beyond the illness she was going through, she found great relief:

> *I felt connected to people, to the world, and surrounded by love. There was a window in my room. I could overhear children's voices. I looked at the sky. I felt connected to life itself and knew that were I to die, life would continue. Being mindful allowed me that perspective.*

Mindfulness involves working with the mind, not battling against it. So rather than saying, "Don't think about illness," say, "If you find yourself thinking about illness, come back to where you are and who you are with, let go of difficulties that have been and gone, and step back from anxiety about catastrophes that haven't even happened." Adopting these attitudes involves a decision, and also a regular practice.

Creating the best environment for healing rather than finding a cure becomes the objective. Even in the midst of serious illness, we can be aware that there are still more things right with us than wrong with us. In connecting to our bodies in this way, we can make sure we benefit as much as possible from the medical interventions, and allow ourselves to stay connected with things that give our lives meaning, even in the midst of discomfort and suffering.

Massage and Cancer Treatment

Delphine de Jong
Remedial Massage Therapist and Oncology Massage Therapist
Diploma of Remedial Massage, Certificate of Oncology Massage

Many people going through cancer treatment seek out massage therapy to relax and make them feel better. It is important to choose a therapist who is experienced and qualified in massaging people with cancer to avoid any complications.

ONCOLOGY MASSAGE

Oncology Massage is specifically tailored massage for people with cancer or a history of cancer. It can enhance physical, emotional and mental relaxation, providing an improved quality of life and greater sense of wellbeing. Oncology massage can also assist with more specific problems such as muscular pain, nerve pain and numbness, release of scar tissue, constipation, and decreased range of motion. Some people find they also experience better sleep and have less fatigue, anxiety and depression. In a clinical world of treatments involving tests, surgeries, chemotherapy and radiotherapy, oncology massage is one treatment that does not cause pain or discomfort and is performed in a caring, nurturing and mindful environment. Oncology massage can be given before, during or after other cancer treatments.

MANUAL LYMPHATIC DRAINAGE

Manual lymphatic drainage can be used to assist people who have compromised lymphatic circulation due to surgery, lymph node removal or limited mobility. It is a very gentle form of massage that helps to return lymphatic fluid from the lymphatic system back into the general circulation for cleansing through the liver and kidneys. This is very important during cancer treatment as the lymphatic fluid is vital in removing the debris of destroyed cells after chemotherapy and radiotherapy. It is also home to many of the immune cells of the body and therefore immune function is improved when lymphatic drainage is at its best.

Surgery and lymph node removal can cause blockages in lymphatic flow, which means fluid may build up and cause swelling, also known as lymphoedema. This can be improved with manual lymphatic drainage, however there is a risk of worsening the condition if the fluid is massaged in the wrong direction. Lymphodema practitioners and therapists trained in complex remedial therapy specialise in redirecting the flow of lymph away from the compromised site, thus reducing the risk.

Appendix

LOW REACTIVE DIET

If you are finding that your digestive system is not coping with food, consider the following suggestions which are designed to reduce foods that are commonly reactive and difficult to digest, and increase nutritious foods that support digestion. Digestive system sensitivities may present as alterations in taste or appetite, heartburn, abdominal pain or cramping, bloating, constipation or diarrhoea.

Vegetables

Include
A large range of fresh vegetables, the more colours the better except those on the avoid list. Organic vegetables are best, as they contain more nutrients and are chemical free. Locally grown are often fresher as they can be bought closer to the time that they are picked. Prepare vegetables in a salad or by lightly steaming them. Vegetable juices can be great way to increase the number of vegetables in your diet, especially when your appetite is reduced.

Avoid
Starchy vegetables including potato and vegetables from the nightshade family if you have a known sensitivity to them. The nightshade family includes potato, eggplant, tomatoes and capsicum. Avoid vegetables that are prepared with cream or are deep-fried. Overcooking takes away many of the vegetable's nutrients.

Fruit

Include

Fresh fruits, preferably organic, as it will be higher in nutrients and is grown without pesticides, herbicides and fungicides. Locally produced food is always better when available, as it hasn't been kept in storage for transportation.

Avoid

The sugar in soft drinks and sugared fruit juices does not come with the fibre contained in the whole fruit. Without the fibre, the sugars are more likely to impact negatively on blood sugar regulation in the body. Also avoid citrus and strawberries if you are sensitive to these. If you feel you are reactive to any other fruits, see a naturopath to establish why.

Nuts, seeds, oils

Include

Nuts including almonds, walnuts, pecans and cashews. Seeds including sesame seeds, pumpkin seeds, linseeds and sunflower seeds have an excellent nutritional profile. Cold pressed oils of olive, sunflower, flaxseed and grape seed are all beneficial.

Avoid

Peanuts have little nutritional value and are best avoided. Also avoid margarine, and oils that are stored in clear plastic containers such as vegetable oil, peanut oil and canola oil. Nuts and seeds are best before roasting and salting.

Grains

Include

Rice (brown or basmati), millet, buckwheat, quinoa, corn, rye, and oats. These may be taken as porridge, bread, crisp bread, cereals or in their basic form to accompany other foods.

Avoid

Bread and bread products made from wheat flour, especially white bread, pasta, cakes, pastries and biscuits as these contain few nutrients and can cause inflammation in the gut and trigger further inflammation throughout the body.

Dairy products

Include

Alternatives to dairy: rice milk, soy milk, coconut milk, almond milk or oat milk.

Avoid

Cow's milk, reduce fat dairy products, cream, cheese, flavored yoghurt and ice cream.

Meat, fish, poultry, pulses

Include

Skinless chicken breast, lamb, salmon, tuna, pulses such as lentils, chickpeas and beans (rinse, cook and chew pulses well). Use organic meats where possible, as these are grown without chemicals and hormones.

Avoid

Beef, veal, cold cuts, tinned meat, ham, sausage, bacon and pork as these contain saturated fat that creates inflammation in sensitive digestive systems. Also avoid eggs for a period of time until you are confident you are not reacting to them. See a naturopath to establish any unclear food allergies or intolerances.

Beverages

Include

Drink plenty of water, herbal tea and vegetable juices. Fruit juices are best consumed moderately, and diluted with water.

Avoid

Coffee, tea, alcohol, soft drinks and diet soft drinks should be avoided. These increase fluid loss from the body and cause stress to the adrenal glands.

Further Reading

Boericke, William. *New manual of homeopathic material media and repertory*, New Delhi: B. Jain Publishers, 2003.

Boger, Cyrus Maxwell. *Boenninghausen's Characteristics Materia Medica and Repertory*, New Delhi: B.Jain Publishers, 1993.

Bone, Kerry & Mills, Simon. *Principles & Practice of Phytotherapy Clinical Guide to Blending Liquid Herbs*, Missouri USA: Churchill Livingstone, 2013.

Braun, Lesley & Cohen, Mark. *Herbs & Natural Supplements,* Vol I & II, 4th Edition. Chatswood: Churchill Livingstone, 2011.

Chancellor, Phillip M. *Illustrated Handbook of the Bach Flower Remedies*, Great Britain: The C. W. Daniel Company, 1971.

Dr. Edward Bach Centre. *The Bach Flower Remedies*, New Canaan, Connecticut: Keats Pub, 1997.

Fritz, Sandy. *Mosby's Fundamentals of Therapeutic Massage* 5th edition, Missouri, USA: Mosby, 2012.

Morrison, Roger M.D. *Desktop Guide To Keynotes and Confirmatory Symptoms*, California: Hahnemann Clinic Publishing, 1993.

Osiecki, Henry. *Cancer, The Importance of Clinical Nutrition in Prevention and Treatment*, Eagle Farm, Australia: Bio Concepts, 2012.

Osiecki, Henry. *The Physician's Handbook of Clinical Nutrition* 7th edition. Eagle Farm, Australia: Bio Concepts, 2006.

Pitchford, Paul. *Healing with Whole Foods* 3rd edition. California, USA: North Atlantic Books, 2002.

Sheffer, Mechthild. *Bach Flower Therapy*, Wellingborough, Northamptonshire: Thorsons 1987.

Trickey, Ruth. *Women, Hormones and the Menstrual Cycle,* Melbourne: Elsevier, 2011.

Whitney, Ellie & Rolfes, Sharon. *Understanding Nutrition* 13th edition. California, USA: Thomson Wadsworth, 2012.

Woodruff, Roger. *Cancer Pain.* Melbourne, Australia: Asperula, 2013.

Endnotes

1   L. Braun & M. Cohen, *Herbs & Natural Supplements* 3rd ed (Chatswood: Churchill Livingstone, 2011).

2   B. Daniele et al, "Oral Glutamine in the Prevention of Fluorouracil Induced Intestinal Toxicity: a Double Blind, Placebo Controlled, Randomised Trial," *Gut* 48 (2001): 28-33; E. Topkan, "Influence of Oral Glutamine Supplementation on Survival Outcomes of Patients Treated with Concurrent Chemoradiotherapy for Locally Advanced Non-Small Cell Lung Cancer," *BMC Cancer* 12(502) (2012), doi 10.1186/1471-2407-12-502.

3   S. Amara, "Oral Glutamine for the Prevention of Chemotherapy-Induced Peripheral Neuropathy," *Annals Pharmacotherapy* Oct;42(10) (2008), doi:10.1345/aph.1L179; W. S. Wang et al, "Oral Glutamine is Effective for Preventing Oxaliplatin-Induced Neuropathy in Colorectal Cancer Patients," *Oncologist* 2007 Mar;12(3) (2007), 312-9.

4   Specific studies have shown the essential fatty acids EPA and DHA found in fish oil increase the response rate to chemotherapy and improved patient survival (A. Laviano et al, "Omega-3 Fatty Acids in Cancer," *Current Opinion In Clinical Nutritional and Metabolic Care* March (2013), doi: 10.1097/MCO.0b013e32835d2d99).

5   DHA particularly has been shown to increase the sensitivity of cancer cells to chemotherapy without increasing damage to healthy cells (N. Hajjaji & P. Bougnoux, "Selective Sensitization of Tumors to Chemotherapy by Marine-Derived Lipids: A Review," *Cancer Treatment Reviews* 39 (2013), 473-88). Concern has been raised that two compounds found in fish oil may cause resistance to chemotherapy (J. M. Roodhart et al, "Mesenchymal Stem Cells Induce Resistance to Chemotherapy

through the Release of Platinum-Induced Fatty Acids," *Cancer Cell* 20 (3) (2011), 370, doi: 10.1016/j.ccr.2011.08.010). Although this certainly warrants further investigation, such compounds are only found in small amounts in fish oil (0%-1.56% of the total lipids) (V. C. Vaughan, M-R Hassing & P A Lewandowski, "Marine Polyunsaturated Fatty Acids and Cancer Therapy", *British Journal of Cancer*, 108(3) (2013), doi: 10.1038/bjc.2012.586) and the suggestion contradicts the body of published literature that demonstrates the benefits of combining fish oil with chemotherapy (R. A. Murphy et al "A Fishy Conclusion Regarding N-3 Fatty Acid Supplementation in Cancer Patients" *Clinical Nutrition* 32(3) (2012), doi: 10.1016/j.clnu.2012.05.013).

[6] R. Raghu Nadhanan et al, "Fish Oil in Comparison to Folinic Acid or Protection Against Adverse Effects of Methotrexate Chemotherapy on Bone," *Journal of Orthopaedic Research* Dec 17 (2013), doi: 10.1002/jor.22565.

[7] ibid.

[8] B. Davis & P. Kris-Etherton, "Achieving Optimal Essential Fatty Acid Status in Vegetarians: Current Knowledge and Practical Implications," *American Journal of Clinical Nutrition* 78(3 Suppl) (2003): 640S-643S.

[9] ibid.

[10] Raghu Nadhanan et al, "Fish Oil in Comparison to Folinic."

[11] ibid.

[12] H. H. Mansour, H. F. Hafez & N. M. Fahmy, "Silymarin Modulates Cisplatin-Induced Oxidative Stress and Hepatotoxicity in Rats," *Journal of Biochemistry and Molecular Biology* 39(6) (2006): 656-61; D. Sadava & S. E. Kane, "Silibinin Reverses Drug Resistance in Human Small-Cell Lung Carcinoma Cells," *Cancer Letters* 333(1) (2013) doi: 10.1016/j.canlet.2013.07.017; A. Rašković et al, "The Protective Effects of Silymarin Against Doxorubicin-Induced Cardiotoxicity and Hepatotoxicity in Rats," *Molecules* 16(10) (2011) doi: 10.3390/molecules16108601.

[13] H. R. Chang et al, "Silibinin Inhibits The Invasion And Migration Of Renal Carcinoma 786-O Cells *In Vitro*, Inhibits The Growth of Xenografts *In Vivo* and Enhances Chemosensitivity to 5-Fluorouracil and Paclitaxel," *Molecular Carcinogenesis* 50(10) (2011) doi: 10.1002/mc.20756; C. Ninsontia et al, "Silymarin Selectively Protects Human Renal Cells from Cisplatin-Induced Cell Death," *Pharmaceutical Biology* 49(10) (2011) doi: 10.3109/13880209.2011.568506.

14   W. H. Paik et al, "Chemosensitivity Induced by Down-Regulation of Microrna-21 in Gemcitabine-Resistant Pancreatic Cancer Cells by Indole-3-Carbinol," *Anticancer Research* 33(4) (2013), 1473-81; B. Cevatemre et al, "Combination of Fenretinide and Indole-3-Carbinol results in Synergistic Cytotoxic Activity inducing Apoptosis against Human Breast Cancer Cells *In Vitro*," *Anticancer Drugs* 24(6) (2013), 577-86, doi: 10.1097/CAD.0b013e328360a921.

15   D. Malejka-Giganti et al, "Suppression of Mammary Gland Carcinogenesis by Post-Initiation Treatment of Rats with Tamoxifen or Indole-3-Carbinol or Their Combination," *European Journal of Cancer Prevention* 16(2) (2007), 130-41.

16   N. Obi et al, "The use of Herbal Preparations to Alleviate Climacteric Disorders and Risk of Postmenopausal Breast Cancer in a German Case-Control Study," *Cancer Epidemiology, Biomarkers & Prevention* 18(8) (2009), 2207-2213.

17   H. H. Henneike-von Zepelin et al, "Isopropanolic Black Cohosh Extract and Recurrence-Free Survival after Breast Cancer," *International Journal of Clinical Pharmacology and Therapeutics* 45(3) (2007), 143-54.

18   H. Fritz, "Black Cohosh and Breast Cancer," *Integrative Cancer Therapies* 13(1) (2014) doi: 10.1177/1534735413477191; R. Walji et al, "Black Cohosh (Cimicifuga racemosa [L.] Nutt.): Safety and Efficacy for Cancer Patients," *Support Cancer Care* 15(8) (2007), 913-21.

19   Braun & Cohen, *Herbs & Natural Supplements*.

20   K. I. Block et al, "Impact of Antioxidant Supplementation on Chemotherapeutic Efficacy: A Systematic Review of the Evidence from Randomized Controlled Trials," *Cancer Treatment Reviews* 33 (2007), 407-18; R. Trickey, *Women, Hormones and the Menstrual cycle* (Melbourne: Elsevier, 2011).

21   L. N. Alschuler & K. Gazella, *The Definitive Guide to Cancer* 3rd ed. (Berkeley: Celestial Arts, 2010).

22   Block et al, "Impact of antioxidant supplementation."

23   M. Fisher & L. X. Lang, "Anticancer Effects and Mechanisms of Polysaccharide-K (PSK): Implications of Cancer Immunotherapy," *Anticancer Research* 22(3) (2002), 1737-54.

24   M. Ghoneum, "Modified Arabinoxylan from Rice Bran, MGN-3/Biobran, Sensitizes Metastatic Breast Cancer Cells to Paclitaxel *In Vitro*,"*Anticancer Research* 34 (2014), 81-7; S. Gollapudi & M. Ghondeum, "MGN-3/Biobran, Modified Arabinoxylan from

Rice Bran, Sensitizes Human Breast Cancer Cells to Chemotherapeutic Agent, Daunorubicin," *Cancer Detection and Prevention* 32 (2008), 1-6.

25   X. Y. Huang, S. Z. Zhang & W. X. Wang, "Enhanced Antitumor Efficacy with Combined Administration of Astragalus and Pterostilbene for Melanoma," *Asia Pacific Journal of Cancer Prevention* 15(3) (2014), 1163-9; H. He et al, "Does the Course of Astragalus-containing Chinese Herbal Prescriptions and Radiotherapy benefit to Non-Small-Cell Lung Cancer Treatment: A Meta-Analysis of Randomised Trials," *Evidence-Based Complementary and Alternative Medicine* (2013), doi: 10.1155/2013/426207; Braun & Cohen, *Herbs & Natural Supplements.*

26   E. Lecumberri et al, "Green Tea Polyphenol Epigallocatechin-3-Gallate (EGCG) as Adjuvant in Cancer Therapy," *Clinical Nutrition* 32(6) (2013), 894-903.

27   E. B. Golden et al, "Green Tea Polyphenols Block the Anticancer Effects Of Bortezomib And Other Boronic Acid-Based Proteasome Inhibitors," *Blood* 113(23) (2009), doi: 10.1182/blood-2008-07-171389.

28   Trickey, *Women, Hormones and the Menstrual cycle.* Soy contains compounds called isoflavones, which have both oestrogen-like and anti-oestrogen effects in the body (X. O. Shu et al, "Soy Food Intake and Breast Cancer Survival," *The Journal of the American Medical Asssociation* 302(22) (2009), 2437-43). These have been investigated for their cancer-protective effects, initially because the high soy-consuming Asian population were found to have less occurance of breast and prostate cancer (H. Yu et al, "Comparative Epidemiology of Cancers of the Colon, Rectum, Prostate and Breast in Shanghai, China versus the United States," *International Journal Epidemiology* 20(1) (1991), 76-81.)

29   Shu et al, "Soy Food Intake."

30   Shu et al, "Soy Food Intake."

31   Despite early conflicting test tube and animal research on soy isoflavones, longer term human studies now show that soy food and soy milk extracts are safe in patients with cancer (Trickey, *Women, Hormones and the Menstrual cycle.*). Except in hypothyroidism, soy isoflavone products do not appear to have any negative effects, however whole soy foods such as soy milk, tofu, soy textured protein foods and soy flour have the most protective effects, as compared to soy supplements made from soy isolates (Shu et al, "Soy Food Intake"). There is also specific research suggesting that prostate cancer recurrence is not increased

by soy consumption (Y. Morimoto et al, "Urinary Estrogen Metabolites During a Randomized Soy Trial," *Nutrition and Cancer* 64(2) (2012), 307-14. doi: 10.1080/01635581.2012.648819).

32 N. Tacyildiz et al, "Soy Isoflavones ameliorate the adverse effects of chemotherapy in children," *Nutrition and Cancer* 62(7) (2010), 1001-5, doi: 10.1080/01635581.2010.509841.

33 Shu et al, "Soy Food Intake."

34 Shu et al, "Soy food intake"; Morimoto et al, "Urinary Estrogen."

35 P. J. Hodges & P. C. A. Kam, "The Peri-Operative Implications of Herbal Medicines," *Anaesthesia* 57 (2002), 889-99. One small study showed that herbal supplements do not alter platelet function, as compared to aspirin (B. W. Beckert et al, "The Effect of Herbal Medicines on Platelet Function: an *In Vivo* Experiment and Review of the Literature," *Plastic and Reconstructive Surgery* 120(7) (2007), 2044-50).

36 Hodges & Kam, "The Peri-Operative Implications."

37 B. Ristow., "Preoperative Use of Alpha Tocopherol Does Not Increase the Risk of Hematoma in the Face Lift Patient: A Preliminary Report," *Plastic and Reconstructructive Surgery*, (2009), 124(5), 1696-9.

38 W. S. Harris, "Expert Opinion: Omega-3 Fatty Acids and Bleeding-Cause for Concern?" *The American Journal of Cardiology*," 99(6A) (2007), 44C-46C. Epub 2006 Nov 29; C. K. Kepler et al, "Omega-3 and Fish Oil Supplements do not cause Increased Bleeding during Spinal Decompression Surgery," *Journal of Spinal Disorders & Techniques* 25(3) (2012), 129-32. doi: 10.1097/BSD.0b013e3182120227; W. S. Harris et al, "Omega- 3 Fatty Acids and Coronary Heart Disease Risk: Clinical and Mechanistic Perspectives," *Atherosclerosis* 197(1) (2008), 12-24; A. C. Salisbury et al, "Relation between Red Blood Cell Omega-3 Fatty Acid Index and Bleeding during Acute Myocardial Infarction," *The American Journal of Cardiology* 109(1) (2012), 13-8; P. D. Watson et al, "Comparison of Bleeding Complications with Omega-3 Fatty Acids and Aspirin and Clopidogrel versus Aspirin and Clopidogrel in Patients with Cardiovascular Disease," *The American Journal of Cardiology* 104(8) (2009), 1052-4; M. Veljovic et al, "Effect of Pretreatment with Omega-3 Polyunsaturated Fatty Acids on Hematological Parameters and Platelets Aggregation in Patients during Elective Coronary Artery

Bypass Grafting," *Military-Medical and Pharmaceutical Review* 70(4) (2013), 396-402.

[39] S. M. He et al, "Effects of Herbal Products on the Metabolism and Transport of Anticancer Agents," *Expert Opinion on Drug Metabolism & Toxicology* 6(10) (2010), 1195-213. doi: 10.1517/17425255.2010.510132.

[40] B. J. Gurley, E. K. Fifer & Z. Gardner, "Pharmacokinetic Herb-Drug Interactions (Part 2): Drug Interactions Involving Popular Botanical Dietary Supplements and Their Clinical Relevance," *Planta Medica* 78(13) (2012), 1490-1514, doi: 10.1055/s-0031-1298331.

[41] A. Sparreboom, M. C. Cox, M. R. Acharya & W. D. Figg, "Herbal Remedies in the United States: Potential Adverse Interactions with Anticancer Agents," *Journal of Clinical Oncology* 22(12) (2004), 2489-503; M. Unger & A. Frank, "Simultaneous Determination of the Inhibitory Potency of Herbal Extracts on the Activity of Six Major Cytochrome P450 Enzymes using Liquid Chromatography/ Mass Spectrometry and Automated Online Extraction," *Rapid Communication in Mass Spectrometry* 18(19) (2004), 2273-81.

[42] Trickey, *Women, Hormones and the Menstrual Cycle.*

[43] E. B. Golden et al, "Green Tea Polyphenols Block the Anti-Cancer Effects of Bortezomib and other Boronic Acid-Based Proteasome Inhibitors,"*Blood* 113(23) (2009), 5927-37.

[44] Y. J. Wu, L.L. Muldoon & E.A. Neuwelt, "The Chemoprotective Agent N-acetylcysteine Blocks Cisplatin-Induced Apoptosis through Caspase Signalling Pathway," 312(2) (2005), 424-31.

[45] Alschuler & Gazella, *The Definitive Guide to Cancer.*

[46] ibid.

[47] V. C. Vaughan, M-R Hassing & P A Lewandowski, "Marine Polyunsaturated Fatty Acids and Cancer Therapy," *British Journal of Cancer,* 108(3) (2013), doi: 10.1038/ bjc.2012.586.